KETO BREAD

The Ultimate Ketogenic Diet Book for Low Carbohydrate; To Enhance Weight Loss, Fat Burning, Promote A Healthy, Easy and Quick to Follow Guides; Recipes

I0463013

By

Emy Skye

CONTENTS

WHY YOU SHOULD
READ THIS BOOK

The KETO BREAD BOOK is a MUST HAVE - an ABSOLUTE MUST HAVE - for all families, careers and associated professionals who need a thorough understanding of the Keto bread and its application for helping reduce fat and some other neurological conditions.

We want to give a clearer picture of what your body will be going through while on the cyclical ketogenic diet. This book will focus on ketosis and what benefits it provides you.

Ketosis is a state in which your body goes on fat burning autopilot. How's that! The fat that is stored in your body begins to get used as energy which will allow for weight reduction of fat, not water or muscle.

Many diets promoted are calorie restriction diets. They help you lose weight, but, most of the weight is in the form of water and muscle. Little fat stores are broken down. Here is the problem with a calorie restrictive eating program. Your metabolism gets

1

slower because your body begins to think it is starving and must slow down the process of losing calories. A slow metabolism equals slower weight loss and faster weight gain!

The cyclical ketogenic diet restricts carbohydrates. By restricting carbohydrates, but, maintaining caloric consumption, your body will have only one option of fuel consumption. That is fat; which is what ketosis is. You are essentially turning on your fat burning machine. Ketones are sent out of your body and fat loss becomes profound. How does this happen? The largest internal organ in your body is the key player. Your liver. The liver has the job of converting fat into ketones. These ketones are then excreted out of the body, weight/fat loss. This is a natural process.

Ketones are created in the liver and are an efficient source of energy for the body. Fatty acids that are broken down from body fat are created in the liver as these ketones. Ketones can only be made present when there is a lack of sugar and glucose in the body. Carbohydrates contain both of these substances. It will always be difficult to lose weight on a high carbohydrate based diet. On the ketogenic diet, the amount of sugar and glucose is reduced to the point where they are no longer the primary source of fuel to be burned in the bloodstream.

We should take a moment and talk about a couple of

myths surrounding the ketogenic diet and whether it is healthy long term. Our bodies can perform in the state of ketosis and be healthy. This state of ketosis is a natural occurrence when the body is not using sugar and glucose. The human body has no problem operating in this state naturally. In other words, it is safe to burn the fat!!

How do you know if you are in a fat burning state? A simple walk to the drug store can answer that quickly. You can use ketone testing strips to check your level of ketosis. Simply capture a urine sample on the strips and check for a color change. The magic color to look for is a pink to purple result. Check the color scale to see your ketone level and where you are in the fat burning zone.

The use of these strips will be your source of the level of ketones being released. This is the gauge by which you will know if you are properly keeping your carbohydrate intake to the necessary level to facilitate ketosis. Don't worry if you are not at the dark purple level. Different people have different levels. Just watch the scale and if you are losing weight, you are pretty much ok!

Here is a word of warning about dehydration. If you are seeing dark purple consistently, please make sure you are drinking enough water. Sometimes the dark purple indicates dehydration. Make sure you keep yourself hydrated properly when on the ketogenic plan.

The fat burning mechanism associated with ketosis is at the heart of the cyclical ketogenic diet. Restricting the carbohydrates and allowing your body the ability to burn those fat reserves will help you achieve your weight loss goals and body contour you have set goals to have. Get your ketone strips and watch your fat burning begin.

INTRODUCTION

For the best diet to rapidly burn fat using the body's natural metabolism, consider a ketogenic diet plan. Nutrition has the strongest effect on the body's production of important hormones, which regulate metabolism and allow the body to burn fat for energy and retain muscle mass, with little need for excessive exercise.

What is a ketogenic diet plan?

Basically, it is a diet that causes the body to enter a state of ketosis. Ketosis is a natural and healthy metabolic state in which the body burns its own stored fat (producing ketones), instead of using glucose (the sugars from carbohydrates found in the Standard American Diet - SAD).

Metabolically speaking, ketogenic foods are very powerful. The amazing benefit is that these foods are also delicious, natural whole foods that are extremely healthy for you.

So what foods are encouraged?

Some of the best-tasting, most fulfilling foods are part of this plan, including lean meats like beef and chicken, healthy sources of protein and high-quality fats like eggs, butter, olive oil, coconut oil and avocado. Also, delicious leafy-green vegetables like kale, chard, and spinach, as well as cruciferous vegetables like broccoli, cabbage and cauliflower.

These foods can be combined with seeds, nuts, sprouts, and a wide range of other amazing foods that lead to incredible health benefits that give your body the protein, healthy fats, and nutrients it needs while providing metabolism-boosting meals for easy cooking at home or on the go.

What foods should be limited?

On a ketogenic diet plan, the main foods to avoid are those high in carbohydrates, sugars, and the wrong types of fats. These foods can be toxic to the body and create excess glucose levels that the body turns into stored fat. These foods increase the level of insulin and blood sugar in the body, and will prevent fat loss even if you are putting a lot of energy into exercise. To avoid these foods, limit your intake of grains, processed foods, vegetable oils (canola, corn, soybean, etc.), milk, margarine, and other high-carbohydrate, high-sugar foods.

But aren't fats bad for you?

We have been told for decades that calories from fats should be reduced to encourage weight loss, but this is a vast over-simplification (still supported by government and industrial food interests) that is no longer accurate according our modern understanding of human nutrition. The reality is that certain fats are not good for you (those high in omega-6 fatty acids), because your body has a hard time processing them. Other fats, particularly medium chain triglycerides (MCTs), are extremely beneficial for weight loss, brain cell generation, and nutrients. These healthy saturated fats should be increased to give your body the energy it needs while in ketosis, while limiting the detrimental trans-fats found in many processed foods.

CHAPTER 1

WHAT ARE THE BENEFITS OF A KETOGENIC DIET PLAN?

- ✓ Burn Stored Fat - By cutting out the high levels of carbohydrates in your diet that produce glucose (sugar), a ketogenic diet plan tells your body to burn stored fat by converting this fat into fatty acids and ketone bodies in the liver. These ketone bodies replace the role of glucose that was being filled by carbohydrates in the diet. This leads to a rapid reduction in the amount of fat stored in the body.

- ✓ Retain Muscle Mass - By including the right fats in your diet, a ketogenic diet plan provides your body with the energy it needs to convert existing fat stores into useful sugars and ketones (through gluconeogenesis), which are an essential source of energy for the brain, muscles, and heart. This has the added benefit of preserving muscle mass, because the healthy fat in the diet gives the body the energy it needs without having to tap into muscle protein to create more sugar. This creates the best of both worlds - burn fat while maintaining muscle mass!

✓ Eliminate Excess Fat - Even better, if your body creates too many ketone bodies by converting existing fat, it will simply eliminate those ketones as a waste product, which means you will basically pee out unwanted body fat!

✓ Reduce Appetite - Lastly, by regulating the powerful metabolic hormones in your body, a ketogenic diet plan will actually reduce your appetite. By lowering your body's insulin resistance and increasing ketones, you will actually feel less hungry on this diet, which is an amazing advantage over other low-calorie, carbohydrate-rich weight loss diets that come with the expectation of lingering hunger.

Start burning fat today without more exercise! Take control of your metabolism naturally by adopting a ketogenic diet plan. Your body was designed for this style of nutrition. Your metabolic state can be optimized by consuming the (delicious) foods that our genetic forefathers thrived on, and this does not include carbohydrate-rich, processed foods loaded with sugars and bad fats. It involves a luxurious and fulfilling diet based on bountiful foods from paleolithic times, including lean meats, vegetables, nuts and seeds, and healthy fats that your body will thank you for.

The main focus to answer what is ketogenic diet lies in the intake and processing of carbohydrates in the diet. Though numbers vary in comparison with body weight, activity level, and mass, a meal plan consisting of less than 60 grams of carbohydrates a day can be considered at ketogenic. This level of crab intake will increase the process of ketosis, allowing for healthier forms of energy production and usage.

When using a ketogenic diet, your body becomes more of a fat-burner than a carbohydrate-dependent machine. Several researches have linked the consumption of increased amounts of carbohydrates to development of several disorders such as diabetes and insulin resistance.

By nature, carbohydrates are easily absorbable and therefore can be also be easily stored by the body. Digestion of carbohydrates starts right from the moment you put them into your mouth.

As soon as you begin chewing them, amylase (the enzymes that digest carbohydrate) in your saliva is already at work acting on the carbohydrate-containing food.

In the stomach, carbohydrates are further broken down. When they get into the small intestines, they are then absorbed into the bloodstream. On getting to the bloodstream, carbohydrates generally increase the blood sugar level.

This increase in blood sugar level stimulates the immediate release of insulin into the bloodstream. The higher the increase in blood sugar levels, the more the amount of insulin that is release.

Insulin is a hormone that causes excess sugar in the bloodstream to be removed in order to lower the blood sugar level. Insulin takes the sugar and carbohydrate that you eat and stores them either as glycogen in muscle tissues or as fat in adipose tissue for future use as energy.

However, the body can develop what is known as insulin resistance when it is continuously exposed to such high amounts of glucose in the bloodstream. This scenario can easily cause obesity as the body tends to quickly store any excess amount of glucose. Health conditions such as diabetes and cardiovascular disease can also result from this condition.

Keto diets are low in carbohydrate and high in fat and have been associated with reducing and improving several health conditions.

One of the foremost things a ketogenic diet does is to

stabilize your insulin levels and also restore leptin signalling. Reduced amounts of insulin in the bloodstream allow you to feel fuller for a longer period of time and also to have fewer cravings.

CHAPTER 2

MEDICAL BENEFITS OF KETOGENIC DIETS

The application and implementation of the ketogenic diet has expanded considerably. Keto diets are often indicated as part of the treatment plan in a number of medical conditions.

Epilepsy

This is basically the main reason for the development of the ketogenic diet. For some reason, the rate of epileptic seizures reduces when patients are placed on a keto diet.

Pediatric epileptic cases are the most responsive to the keto diet. There are children who have experience seizure elimination after a few years of using a keto diet.

Children with epilepsy are generally expected to fast for a few days before starting the ketogenic diet as part of their treatment.

Cancer

Research suggests that the therapeutic efficacy of the ketogenic diets against tumor growth can be enhanced when combined with certain drugs and procedures under a "press-pulse" paradigm.

It is also promising to note that ketogenic diets drive the cancer cell into remission. This means that keto diets "starves cancer" to reduce the symptoms.

Alzheimer Disease

There are several indications that the memory functions of patients with Alzheimer's disease improve after making use of a ketogenic diet.

Ketones are a great source of alternative energy for the brain especially when it has become resistant to insulin. Ketones also provide substrates (cholesterol) that help to repair damaged neurons and membranes. These all help to improve memory and cognition in Alzheimer patients.

Diabetes

It is generally agreed that carbohydrates are the main culprit in diabetes. Therefore, by reducing the amount of ingested carbohydrate by using a ketogenic diet, there are increased chances for improved blood sugar control.

Also, combining a keto diet with other diabetes treatment plans can significantly improve their overall effectiveness.

Gluten Allergy

Many individuals with gluten allergy are undiagnosed with this condition. However, following a ketogenic diet showed improvement in related symptoms like digestive discomforts and bloating.

Most carbohydrate-rich foods are high in gluten. Thus, by using a keto diet, a lot of the gluten consumption is reduced to a minimum due to the elimination of a large variety of carbohydrates.

CHAPTER 3

WHAT IS KETOSIS?

Ketosis is a normal metabolic state of the body when ketones are used as a source of energy instead of glucose. Our body will go into the state of ketosis when there is not enough glucose in the body for the production of energy. In this state, the body will start burning the stored fats that will increase the level of ketones in the blood. These ketones will be used by our brain for the production of energy.

When you first deprive your body of carbohydrates and replace them with protein and fat, the metabolism begins to shift to accommodate this. The first stage is known as lipolysis, and is the initial burning of fat to use as energy.

Ketosis, put simply, is the second part of the process that takes place when your body's metabolism shifts from getting energy from carbohydrates to taking it from fat. When it is taking place, this is the time that you lose the most fat. The name ketosis relates to the blocks fat that are stored for release as energy, which are known as ketones.

Ketosis shouldn't lead to a loss of muscle tissue, unless you are completely out of fat. This makes you even better at burning fat, as you retain the strength throughout your body to do so, particularly in the smaller internal muscles. When ketosis is taking place it is possible to lose up to a stone in little over a week.

The main side effects of ketosis are bad breath and sluggish mobility. Bad breath is caused due to a change in the bacteria and enzymes throughout the digestive system, and slow movement because fat is much harder to use for energy production, making you low on energy. Neither of these are likely to be harmful.

However, if you are diabetic, ketosis can lead to a condition called ketoacidosis, which results in the blood becoming more acidic. This will then cause symptoms including confusion, vomiting, and can even go as far as causing comas and death.

If you want to know if your body is carrying out ketosis, head down to your local chemist and buy ketone testing strips. These operate in a very similar way to universal indicator strips (if you can remember your old chemistry lessons) and will turn purple if ketones are contained in the urine.

If you're thinking about starting a low carb diet then you need to know about ketosis and dieting

There are some individuals who encourage ketosis by following the Ketosis diet, which is a special diet plan. The purpose of this diet is to try to burn all the stored fats in the body by relying on the fatty meals for energy. The amount of carbs in the diet is reduced.

It is a process that is commonly observed in patients suffering from diabetes. When their body does not have enough insulin or they are not using the insulin properly the body will go into ketosis for the production of energy.

CHAPTER 4

INTERESTING FACTS
ABOUT KETOSIS

Carbohydrates are major sources of energy and have some specific roles in the human body. They are the primary sources of fuel for the human brain. Although ketone bodies can supply most of the energy to the brain during a starvation state, the axons cannot use anything but glucose. This makes carbohydrates vital to the function of every single neuron in the brain and in the rest of the nervous system. In addition, carbohydrates are the only sources of fuel that are acceptable to the kidneys and the red blood cells.

Now most people will find the necessity of carbohydrates to the red blood cells to be surprising because the red blood cells carry oxygen. However, their job is to transport the oxygen and not to use it up for themselves so they have to derive their energy from anaerobic glycolysis. However, the brain is by far the largest consumer of carbohydrates. The combination of the brain, kidneys, and red blood cells consume an average of about 130 to 150 grams (~500 to 600 calories) of carbohydrates per day.

If the body is deprived of adequate carbohydrates, it will use the processes of gluconeogenesis (making of new glucose) and ketogenesis (making of ketones) to provide energy for vital functions. It is important to note that fats are not good fuels for making glucose because the glycerol group is the only part of a triglyceride that can be used to manufacture glucose. The fatty acids themselves can only be oxidized or converted to ketones.

A low-carbohydrate diet, along with a high-protein and low-fat diet, has become a part of the strategy devised by most dietitians for losing weight. The main disadvantage of high-carb foods like rice, white bread, and pasta is that it tends to create belly fat that most people find very difficult to get rid of. A low-carb diet helps in reducing the blood pressure and increasing good cholesterol. Another advantage of having a low-carb diet is that it helps reduce the levels of sugar and starch in the body, which in turn helps in losing weight. Over time, such a diet helps in reducing the craving for sugar-based foods like pastries and chocolates.

However, some people mistake a low-carb diet for an

absolutely no-carb diet, which could be dangerous. The human body needs some carbohydrates for energy and for maintaining adequate glucose levels. A no-carbohydrate diet could result in unwanted abnormally low levels of glucose. In countries like India and China, where rice is part of a staple diet, people are advised to lower the intake of such foods, and not totally avoid it.

While bananas and potatoes have the required amount of essential fibers needed for a healthy body, they are very high in carbohydrates. This is why most people on a low-carb diet plan, should avoid bananas and potatoes. There is a popular misconception that low-carb foods lack fiber content. This lacks truth because low-carb vegetables such as broccoli, spinach, and other leafy vegetables have ideal amounts of protein, carbohydrates and fiber. These are also non-starchy unlike potatoes and yam, which have a high content of starch. Some low-carb high protein foods are fish, eggs, lean beef, and lean veal.

People generally tend to cut fruits from their diet to reduce their carb intake, which is a mistake. Other than bananas, most other fruits like blackberries, papaya, strawberry, apples, and oranges are very rich in fiber and contain low levels of starch. Salads, wheat bread, soybeans, brown rice, oat meals, and low-fat dairy products are perfect for a low-carb diet plan.

Almost all body builders and weight lifters have a strict diet high in proteins and hardly any carbohydrates. Here is an interesting fact about Sylvester Stallone. It is believed that while preparing for his well-toned muscled look for the movie First Blood, Sly followed a diet consisting of just egg whites six times a day along with a piece of potato together with daily workouts. During the filming of the movie, he had a little fruit or fresh juice once or twice a week. This diet helped him avoid accumulation of any fat in the body.

However, experts warn that such a diet is not suited for everybody. People who are on a temporary high-protein diet tend to put on too much weight once they get back to their high-carb diet. Some other complications of a very low-carb diet are low blood pressure and ketosis. Ketosis is a condition where the body starts using stored fatty acids, as it does not have the required amount of carbohydrates to use glucose. This affects both the body and the brain negatively in the long run. It is strongly advised that you must consult an expert dietician or your physician who can recommend the right amount of proteins and carbohydrates required, based on the specific needs of the person. Keeping these points in mind can help you meet your health goals effectively and efficiently.

Here are some of the interesting facts about ketosis that you should know about.

The body will go into ketosis when there is not enough glucose in the body for the production of energy.

It is a process in which fats are broken down into ketones for the production of energy.

In order to achieve ketosis, people have to follow a special Ketosis diet in which there is a high amount of fats, adequate proteins and lower level of proteins.

There are many people who are following the Ketosis diet in order to lose some extra weight and maintain their level of energy in a most efficient way.

CHAPTER 5

HOW TO GET INTO
KETOSIS QUICKLY

Test Your Ketones

There are many people who are following a Ketosis diet but the issue is that their body is not in ketosis. This is the reason they are unable to maintain their weight or lose the extra pounds. It is important for you to understand that sometimes even after following the ketogenic diet your body will not undergo ketosis, the reason is that you may be making some serious mistakes. In this situation, it is better that you test the level of ketones in your body on regular basis. That is the only way you can find out whether your body is in ketosis or not.

There are different types of testing methods available that you can use to test the level of ketones in your body. The simplest method is using the strips. You have to urinate on the strips and they will let you know the level of ketones in your body. There are some sugar meters available as well that can provide you accurate results. In case you are confused and it is hard for you to find the accurate results, the best solution would be consulting a doctor. He/she will let you know the tests you should go through to find out whether your body is in ketosis or not.

How to Get into Ketosis Quickly Ketosis is the natural process of the body in which our body will consume the stored fats to produce ketones that will supply energy to all parts of the body including the brain. In order to get and stay in ketosis, you have to increase your fat intake, have moderate proteins and reduce the amount of carb intake. You will be surprised to know that there are some individuals who are having a keto diet but they are unable to get into ketosis. This is the reason that even after maintaining a keto diet they are unable to enjoy the benefits that come with it. You should know that it is important for your body to get into ketosis otherwise you will not be able to lose any weight. Here we have some of the ways you can use to assure that your body will get into ketosis quickly. How to Stay in Ketosis

Before we can share some tips with you to get into ketosis, it is important for you to understand that how you can stay in ketosis. It is important for your internal system to get the signals that you will not get any kind of carbs for a long time. That is how it will make it possible for your body to assure that it will keep using fats to stay in ketosis. It is one of the best ways to assure that you will not let your body get out of ketosis. It will allow you to enjoy your healthy weight once again. Here we have some of the ways you can get into ketosis.

Minimize Your Carb Consumption

If you want to stay in ketosis it is important for you to minimize your carb intake. Before you can start increasing the consumption of fats, it is still important that you first reduce your carb intake. That is the only way you will be able to assure that there are no residuals carbs left in your body that can be used for the production of glucose. It will take your metabolic system towards the consumption of all the stored fats that you have.

Have More Oils in Your Diet

After reducing the carbs, you have to increase the oil intake to get into ketosis. You have to assure that you add more healthy oils to your diet that will help increase the content of fats in your body and help you stay healthy. Some of the healthy oils you can include in your diet are.

Coconut oils

Olive oils

Sunflower oils

The best way to consume this oil is to add more oil while cooking your food. You can have more fried products if you like but assure that you will not use hydrogenated oils because they are not good for your body.

Increase The Healthy Fat Intake

One of the most important things you have to consider to stay in ketosis is to increase your healthy fat intake. There are several food items that will allow you to increase your natural fat intake. It is better that you include healthy food items like fish, meat, fruits, butter, dairy and all other healthy food items that will help you maintain your health. You will have to assure that you take the process slowly because you cannot suddenly move towards the fatty diet.

Add a More Physical Activity

It is important that you add more physical activity to your routine if you want to get into ketosis. Remember that if you are having keto diet but you are not working out or trying to burn your calories than your body into ketosis. The reason is that when your body will not need energy it will not try to convert the fats into ketones. This is the reason that most people cannot get into ketosis. That is why it is better that you include proper physical activity into your life. It will allow you to maintain your physical fitness.

Fasting is a Reliable Solution

One of the most reliable ways to get and stay in ketosis if it is hard for you to add physical activity to your life is by doing fast. There is the option of short and long fast available. The benefit of fasting is that when you will not eat anything for a long time your body will start consuming the stored fats for the production of energy. It will allow you to quickly get into ketosis. However, fasting is a little tough. You have to assure that you are determined to keep your fast because that is the only way you can maintain your health.

Maintain Your Protein Intake

Do not forget to maintain your protein intake when you want to get into ketosis. There are some people who will only pay attention to the balance of fats and carbs that they will forget about their proteins. You should know that if you will not maintain protein intake your muscle mass will be reduced. It is important that you maintain the normal intake of protein because that is the only way you can maintain your muscle mass and assure that you stay healthy.

Listen to Your Body

A common mistake most people make is they do not listen to their body when they want to stay in ketosis. You should know that staying in ketosis does not mean that you should be consuming something all the time. When your body is not hungry and it is telling you to not consume anything, it is better that you do not eat anything. It will allow you to maintain your health in the best possible way. Overconsumption of food will not let your body stay in ketosis and it will become hard for you to lose all the extra pounds. That is why it is important that you respect your appetite.

Go Strictly on Your Diet

It is important that with the passage of time you will have to go strictly on your diet if you want to lose weight and get into ketosis. You should know that after some time your body will get used to the system and it will not stay in ketosis. In this condition, it is better that you consume a strict diet because that is the only way you will be able to maintain your health. You can increase the fats intake, do fasting for a longer duration, add more workout sessions to your routine and assure that you challenge your body to assure that you can stay healthy.

Drink Lots and Lots of Water

If you want to stay in ketosis, it is important that you drink as much water as you can. You should at least drink 10 to 12 glasses of water. It will help you to keep your body hydrated for a long time and you will be able to control your cravings. In this way, you will be able to remove all the toxins from your body and it will allow you to keep your inner systems healthy. Once you start drinking water you will notice that your skin will improve and there are many negative effects in your body that can be stopped with increased consumption of water.

Keto Supplements Can Help

You can consider including keto supplements in your diet if you want to get into ketosis. There are such a large number of new supplements out right now that enable you to go into ketosis truly rapidly and even go astray from an immaculate supper plan. By taking these exogenous items, you will figure out how to get into ketosis in 24 hours.

CHAPTER 6

DO'S AND DON'T'S OF
KETOSIS WEIGHT LOSS

Many diet plans and weight loss programs fail to achieve stabile, low-risk and healthy weight loss. Why is that? Several factors may be identified, such as insufficient professional feedback for diet plans, inappropriate carbs/fats/protein ratio, or some facts concerning individual features of each person's metabolism. But, one specific weight loss and diet program found its way to the top thanks to its efficiency and health-friendly orientation. It's a ketosis weight loss program, one of the most recent weight loss programs designed specifically to achieve the best possible results. You shouldn't jump into conclusion that the ketosis weight loss program is some miracle which absorbs fats from our body and gives us the perfect figure we wanted. It's not that simple, and as with every other diet plan you should follow some guidelines that will help you increase the effects of ketosis weight loss program. Here they're presented as do's and don't's.

Do's:

Follow the ketosis weight loss program as indicated since that can only guarantees you adequate results. It shouldn't be so hard, especially when you see. That only after a week or two your body starts losing a significant amount of fat!

Ketosis weight loss implies strictly designed diet plan, consisting of high-fat/adequate-protein/low-curb leverage. That means, if you stick up to this leverage, you should run into ketosis weight loss program in no time!

Before you start with the ketosis weight loss program you should consult with a nutritionist or dietician. The main reason is that this diet plan is radical, causing some more or less severe side-effects such as fatigue, headache, faints and so forth.

Don'ts:

Do not modify any aspect of the ketosis weight loss program. The calculations of fat/carbs/protein ratio is precise and specific, based on numerous researches and the long medical history of the diet. So, modifying anything from the ketosis weight loss plan may indicate inadequate results.

Avoid carbs as long as you can, even if you are granted permission to use them after app. A month of using the ketosis weight loss program. The carbs are the major maleficent to human metabolism, causing severe health issues such as diabetes.

Do not cheat on the diet plan! There are thousands and thousands of recipes you could use in your ketosis weight loss program so there is no excuse for abandoning the program because ingredients repeat itself. Use your creativity and try to find the combination it suits you.

WHAT CAN YOU EAT ON A KETOGENIC DIET?

Fat shedding diets are the most basic way to turn when you are desperate to ditch a couple of pounds. Reducing fat can be truly complex. Low calorie diet plans develop the loss of meat bulk in addition to fat. In cases like this if we beat down muscle our metabolic rate gets smaller. Needless to mention a fall in metabolism normally to make weight-loss more exhausting.

Defined weight loss arrangements are more desirable as set side by side with others. Weight burning diets work the best. results With a calorie closed diet computer program our cats are not stimulated to burn up fat. When caloric intake is limited too much our bodies go into a hunger mode.

Other slim down plans that people commonly see early achievement with are no carb diets for instance Atkins. In the majority of these diets show efficiently at lowering weight at first. Regrettably long-term achievement adopting zero carbohydrate diets isn't as beneficial as the actual success found with fantastic fat shedding diets. One of the maximum troubles with this portion of weight-reduction plan is that often after a couple of weeks they will appear to be demanding to stick to. It should to be told that a ketogenic diet may have a lot of overall fitness perks. Ketogenic diet plans were used to deal with various ailments through the generations. The sheer point of a good ketogenic diet tend to be outside of the confines of this column.

Any time you are looking at shedding fat, low fat weight reduction programs aren't very effective either. Healthful fats really are a critical component of weight shedding diets. Oftentimes when you look into the nutrition content associated with low-fat foods there will be sugar added in. Enjoying a diet regime full with sugars is sure to assist you to pack on the fat. Sugar is a low fat food after all. This is generally a major point of failure pertaining to a lot of the well acknowledged diet plans. For all the indicated body weight loss arrangements that contain the point plans, it will be possible to eat just higher sugar meals.

These useless unhealthy calories won't help body weight loss.

What exactly helps make fat burning diets do the job? Successful diets include the correct array of healthful proteins healthy carbs along with healthier fats. They will restrict or remove adverse fats and basic sugars really.

Absorbing more meals per day is really an elementary principal of fat burning diets. To really encourage your metabolism, demolish six meals a day as opposed to three big meals. These are going to be 6 smaller sized grub to keep the metabolism fettered every bit the day.

A ketogenic diet is basically a diet which converts your body from burning sugar to burning fat. Around 99% of the wold's population have a diet which cause their body to burn sugar. As a result, carbohydrates are their primary fuel source used after digesting carbs. This process makes people gain weight, however a diet of fat and ketones will cause weight loss. As you ask what can you eat on a ketogenic diet, first of all eat up to 30 to 50 grams of carbs per day. Next, let us discover more about what you can have on your plate and how the ketogenic diet affects your health.

THE IMPORTANCE OF SUGAR PRECAUTION ON THE KETOGENIC DIET

Keto shifts your body from a sugar burner to a fat burner by eliminating the dietary sugar derived from carbohydrates. The first obvious reduction you should make from your current diet is sugar and sugary foods. Although sugar is a definite target for deletion, the ketogenic diet focuses upon the limitation of carbohydrates. We need to watch out for sugar in a number of different types of foods and nutrients. Even a white potato which is carb-heavy may not taste sweet to your tongue like sugar. But once it hits your bloodstream after digestion, those carbs add the simple sugar known as glucose to your body. The truth is, our body can only store so much glucose before it dumps it elsewhere in our system. Excess glucose becomes what is known as the fat which accumulates in our stomach region, love handles, etc.

PROTEIN AND IT'S PLACE IN KETO

Protein is absolutely required for your body's normal functioning, as it helps synthesize your enzymes and hormones. It maintains your fluid balance and the building of antibodies against infections. It also is the basic building block for your muscles, bones, cartilage, skin, hair and blood, and is essential for the formation of all of the cells in your body You should eat protein-rich foods such as meat, cheese, milk, fish and eggs to get enough protein in your daily diet. You can also find protein in soy products, as well as in combinations of food such as rice or corn with beans, when it comes to vegetable proteins that you may consume.

If you increase protein without adding more calories and exercise to your daily life, instead of building muscle mass you will put your other body systems under undue stress. And eating more protein while increasing calorie intake -- but keeping at the same exercise levels -- builds an equal amount of additional fat and muscle. Meanwhile, a diet where protein is more than 30% of your calorie intake causes a buildup of toxic ketones. A "ketogenic" diet, or one high in ketones, pushes your kidneys to excessively flush themselves free of toxins. This can cause you to lose a significant amount of water, which puts you at serious risk of dehydration, especially if you exercise heavily during your workouts.

Such water loss will make it appear you're losing weight, when in actuality you're not. Plus you will be losing, not gaining, muscle mass and bone calcium from this ketogenic diet, while the stress of dehydration can also badly affect your heart. Dehydration from a ketogenic diet can make you dizzy and weak, give you bad breath, and lead to other health-related problems. This can be the result of a high-protein, low-carb "fad" diet - one that emphasizes proteins excessively.

You should eat a balanced diet rich in fruits, vegetables, whole grains, lean meats, fish and complex carbohydrates, not one heavy in protein alone. But protein is optimal for immune functioning, and you may need heavier amounts of it when injured or otherwise undergoing any serious healing processes.

Proteins are made up of several different amino acids, some of which your body can make on its own. But some of them have to be ingested. These are called the "essential" amino acids. You must eat a variety of foods to make sure you're getting all of your essential amino acids. Lack of these can cause growth failure, loss of muscle mass, decreased immune system functioning, weakening of the circulatory and respiratory systems - and even death.

The most common source of protein in the American diet is meat, but milk and other dairy products are rich in it. To avoid too much fat with your protein, eat leaner cuts of meat, and cook without adding fat by baking, broiling, barbecuing or boiling your meat. By eating beans and lentils as well as a variety of vegetables and grains, you can add terrific sources of vegetable protein to your diet. Nuts and seeds are also great sources of non-animal protein.

The average adult American needs eight grams of protein each day per twenty pounds of normal body weight. Yet we generally eat twice that much protein daily. If you balance your carbohydrates with your proteins, and eat a variety of foods to make sure you get all of the amino acids you need, you will be eating a healthy diet. You should also make sure you keep your diet low in fats, oils and refined sugars. Those substances have no proteins, and hardly any other nutrients, with one gram containing nine calories of energy. You do need some saturated and unsaturated fats in your food, every day. Unfortunately, "junk food" laden American eating habits tend to provide far too much of these fats.

Your daily diet should contain no more than 30% total calories from fats, hopefully far less than that. The upper limit on the amount of fat in your diet will depend on how many calories you need to maintain your weight, and cutting back on fat can help you consume fewer calories. But some dietary fat is needed for good health. It supplies energy and the essential fatty acids, which like the essential amino acids can only be gleaned from your consumption of certain foods. Fats also promote absorption of the fat-soluble vitamins A, D, E and K.

High levels of saturated fat and cholesterol are linked to increased blood cholesterol and put you at risk for heart disease. Fat is also associated with protein-rich food such as meat and dairy products. So you should lower the daily amount of protein and fat that you consume to an acceptable level, while raising the amount of complex carbohydrates you consume to at least 50% of your daily calorie intake. This will ensure that you are eating a proper and not a "fad" -- or risky to your health - diet every day. Eating meals and snacks rich in whole grains, fruits and vegetables, as well as some high protein and certain "fatty" foods, will help you to obtain your desired weight and to keep fit

One source of carbohydrates which some people overlook in their diet is protein. Overconsumption of protein according to the tolerance level of your body will result in weight gain. Because our body converts excess protein into sugar, we must moderate the amount of protein we eat. Moderation of our protein intake is part of how to eat ketogenic and lose weight. First of all, identify your own tolerance of daily protein and use as a guide to maintain an optimal intake of the nutrient. Second, choose your protein from foods such as organic cage-free eggs and grass-fed meats. Finally, create meals in variety that are delicious and maintain your interest in the diet. For instance, a 5 ounce steak and a few eggs can provide an ideal amount of daily protein for some people.

Caloric Intake on The Ketogenic Diet

How many calories should I be eating? How much protein, how much fat, how many carbs? What amount to gain muscle? How much to lose fat?

These are incredibly common questions, but rarely can we find a good answer to them. And unfortunately, this is why so many of us stall in our progress. Inadvertently overeating, or undereating, is a widespread dietary dilemma, and one that could so easily be avoided, with the right information.

Calories are another important consideration for what can you eat on a ketogenic diet. Energy derived from the calories in the food we consume help our body to remain functional. Hence, we must eat enough calories in order to meet our daily nutritional requirements. Counting calories is a burden for many people who are on other diets. But as a ketogenic dieter, you don't have to worry nearly as much about calorie counting. Most people on a low-carb diet remains satisfied by eating a daily amount of 1500-1700 kcals in calories.

Fats, The Good & The Bad

Fat is not bad, in fact many good healthy fats exist in whole foods such as nuts, seeds and olive oil. Healthy fats are an integral part of the ketogenic diet and are available as spreads, snacks and toppings. Misconceptions in regards to eating fat are that a high amount of it is unhealthy and causes weight gain. While both statements are in a sense true, the fat which we consume is not the direct cause of the fat which appears on our body. Rather, the sugar from each nutrient we consume is what eventually becomes the fat on our body.

Balance Your Nutrients Wisely

Digestion causes the sugars we eat to absorb into the bloodstream and the excess amount transfer into our fat cells. High carbohydrate and high protein eating will result in excess body fat, because there is sugar content in these nutrients. So excessive eating of any nutrient is unhealthy and causes weight gain. But a healthy diet consists of a balance of protein, carbohydrates and fats according to the tolerance levels of your body.

Just about everyone can accomplish a ketogenic diet with enough persistence and effort. In addition, we can moderate a number of bodily conditions naturally with keto. Insulin resistance, elevated blood sugar, inflammation, obesity, type-2 diabetes are some health conditions that keto can help to stabilize. Each of these unhealthy conditions will reduce and normalize for the victim who follows a healthy ketogenic diet. Low-carb, high-fat and moderate protein whole foods provide the life-changing health benefits of this diet.

CHAPTER 7

WHAT IS KETOGENIC MEASUREMENT?

Though a dietary plan that follows an established program will in fact lower glucose production, your doctor can evaluate how effective your diet is through a few simple tests.

Though it is not required to know what is ketogenic conditioned leveling in order for a plan to work, you may wish to check to ensure everything is functioning as it should.

How Ketosis Works

The individuals who are interested in starting Ketogenic diet want to know that how this diet plan can help them reduce a reasonable amount of weight. You should know that once the assimilation of fats will start in your body, you will have enough energy that you will not have to feel hungry. It will allow you to stay focused on your work and you will not have to worry about consuming more food. It will allow you to avoid storing more fats in your body. You will notice that your overall health will improve and in the limited time, you will be able to lose all the extra fats that you have stored in your body in a healthy and safe way.

Before you can decide that you would like to follow the process of ketosis it is important for you to understand how ketosis works. That is the only way you will be able to generate the positive results that come with the process. Here are some of the simple steps in which you can get the positive results.

Reduce Carbs

It is important that you reduce the level of glycogen and glucose in your body. Once the level of glucose is depleted only than you will be able to achieve ketosis. In order to make it possible you have to reduce your consumption of carbs. The best way to make it possible is consuming an alternative source of energy that is fats.

HOW MANY CARBS CAN I EAT ON KETO DIET?

Fats Breakdown

Once your body will reach the level of ketosis when

there is no source of glucose available, it will start breaking down the fats. The process of breakdown of fats is known as beta-oxidation. At this stage, the level of acetyl-CoA will increase and it will be converted into acetoacetate. After that conversion of acetoacetate into beta-hydroxybutyrate will cause the production of ketones. These ketone bodies will float around in the blood and provide your brain and body with the required amount of energy.

Ketosis Signs and Symptoms

There are various signs and symptoms of ketosis that will clearly indicate that the level of ketones in your body has increased. Here are some of the common signs and symptoms you need to know about.

You will start losing weight

There will be a loss of appetite and cravings

In the first few weeks of ketosis diet the energy level will decrease but after that energy level will increase

There will be a fruity smell in your breath

There are some individuals who may find it hard to digest fats in the beginning due to which they may have to suffer from constipation or diarrhea.

Importance of Ketosis Diet

Obesity is a common problem in the present age that leads to various other health issues. This is the reason most people are interested in losing all the extra weight in order to maintain their health and assure that they can look good. There are many people who want to know why going on a ketosis diet is important for their health. Here we have some of the reasons why you should be on a ketosis diet.

Weight Loss

There are many people who are interested in losing all the extra weight but they are unable to maintain the weight loss plan. However, the Ketosis Diet will make the entire process simple for them. When you will eat more fats, your appetite will be reduced. It will help you control your craving and you can easily stay hungry for a long time. As well as fats will help burn all the stored fats in your body. It will help you lose all the extra pounds and you will be able to maintain a healthy weight. In this way, you will not have to worry about following a strict diet or exercise plan. You can prepare delicious meals and maintain your weight loss plan with ketosis diet.

The easiest way to burn fat! When your body is in ketosis, it is burning fat cells for energy instead of carbs.

MAINTAIN HIGH ENERGY LEVEL

The biggest attraction of the diet plan is that you will be able to maintain a higher level of energy for a long period of time. When you will start the diet plan in the early stages you might feel tired because your body will take some time to get into ketosis. But once the level of ketones is maintained in your body, you will not have to deal with any issues. Fats have the highest level of energy and once ketones are providing your body will be energy that you need, there is no need to worry about getting tired. It will help increase your stamina and you will not have to deal with any serious issues. You will be able to work out for a long time as well.

The Mental Focus Will Improve

You will be surprised to know that how ketones will help increase your focus. The reason is that when you use glucose as the source of energy, the level of glucose will easily fall down. If you are unable to maintain the level of glucose in your blood, you will start feeling tired and exhausted. Due to which it would get hard for you to maintain your attention and focus on the given task. However, once you are on ketosis you will not have to deal with such issues. Once your brain will get a constant source of energy you will not have to deal with any lower level of energy, so your focus and concentration will be maintained.

DISEASE PREVENTION

One of the best things about ketosis is that it will protect you from various types of diseases. It will help decrease inflammation in the body. Inflammation is the biggest cause of various health issues that we have been dealing with. It will protect you from cancer by helping to maintain the normal division and growth of cells. There are various other health issues that will be prevented once you are on ketosis. It will lower the level of LDL in the blood that will protect you from heart issues. Research has shown that ketosis is also beneficial for seizure. It can help control the seizures.

Physical Performance Will Improve

Once you are on ketosis your overall performance will improve. It will help enhance your endurance. In this way, you can work for long hours without getting tired. You will notice that once you will start working you will ever forget that for how long you have been working. It will get easier for you to complete your tasks in limited time and that is how your performance will improve. In this way, you will play an important role in increasing the productivity of your business or company for which you are working.

It will improve your ranking in the company. You should know that ketosis will help you maintain your health in a natural and healthy way.

Reduce Acne

You may have doubts in mind that when you will start consuming more fats the production of oil will increase, due to which you may have to suffer from pimples and acne. You should know that ketosis can help reduce acne. You should know that one of the major causes of acne in the increased level of sugar and carbs in the blood. It causes the blockage of pores due to which formation of pimples and acne starts. However, once you are on ketosis you will control your consumption of carbs. In this way, the level of sugar in blood will be controlled and you will notice a reduction in acne.

CHAPTER 8

IS KETOSIS DIET HEALTHY AND SAFE FOR EVERYONE?

There are many people who want to know whether ketosis diet is safe and healthy for them or not. They are interested in the process because they want to lose weight but do not know whether it would be the right diet plan or not. No doubt ketosis diet can help lose weight but the long-term effects of being constantly in ketosis have not been properly investigated. However, as a short-term weight loss solution ketosis is very beneficial for people.

There are many individuals who are interested in starting a Ketogenic diet. However, it is important to know there are some restrictions that come with the diet plan. Before we can get started with the explanation of Ketogenic diet, it is important to understand whether you can maintain the diet plan or not.

- You take medications for diabetes like insulin

51

- Taking medication for high blood pressure.

- Breastfeeding your baby.

In case you are dealing with any of these issues or taking other medications, it is better that you consult a professional before starting the Ketogenic diet.

You should know that when you are on a ketosis diet you have to maintain a healthy amount of ketones in your body. High level of ketones in the bloodstream can be really dangerous for you. It can make your blood acidic that is a dangerous medical condition.

Another thing you need to know is that response to ketosis is different in everyone. There are some people in which the body will start producing insulin to slow down the process of production of ketones in order to control the level of toxicity in blood, while others cannot. That is why it is important to monitor the level of ketones in your body because that is the only way you can maintain a normal level of ketones and enjoy the health benefits that come with the process. It is important to know all these while following the ketosis diet.

DANGERS OF THE KETO DIET YOU SHOULD KNOW ABOUT

Many people are worried about their weight. They want to have a perfect figure, but it gets hard for them to follow the exercise plan because they do not have enough time for it. As well as they have to maintain their healthy diet because they cannot compromise on their performance due to which dieting is not an option. In this situation, the best solution that most people have is the keto diet plan. It is a process in which we take our body into the ketosis state by eating more fats and controlling our consumption of carbs and proteins. In this way, our body will consume the stored fats and it will effectively help in the weight loss. No doubt it is effective and beneficial for the health, but there are various dangers of the keto diet that you should know about before getting started with the process.

1. Diarrhea

A common problem that most people have to deal with when they are on a keto diet is diarrhea. The reason is that our body is not used to consuming more fats than carbs. As well as you should know that the breakdown and assimilation of fats takes more time. This is the reason when the body will be unable to digest the fats properly it would lead to some serious digestive issues. It may start with vomiting and nausea feeling, but if you do not pay attention, you may have to suffer from serious diarrhea.

2. Reduced Performance

There are many people who have complained that after following the keto diet their energy level reduced and they were not able to give their best performance. It is the worst dangers of the keto diet because you will not be able to concentrate on the given work when you do not have the level of energy in your body that you need to focus on your work. The ketones produced in the keto diet cannot produce the same amount of energy like the glucose that is why reduced energy is a common issue until your body will get used to the process.

3. Nutritional Deficiency

One of the biggest dangers of the keto diet is that you may have to deal with nutritional deficiency. Most of the food items that you are planning to consume will contain more fats. This is the reason you will not be able to maintain the healthy nutrients in your diet. We all know that deficiency of even a minor nutrient from the diet can lead to various other health issues. That is why while preparing your keto diet plan it is important that you pay proper attention to the nutrients that you will get from your diet.

4. Ketoacidosis

There are many people who suffer from acidosis after following the keto diet. The reason is that ketones produced by the keto diet are acidic in nature. If you maintain the keto diet for a long time the ketones product, used in the body will exceed the normal limit, and they will make the blood acidic. We all know that it is very important to maintain the pH of blood because slightly acidic or basic pH can lead to liver and kidney failure and various other issues. That is why it is advised that we should not maintain the keto diet for a prolonged duration to avoid dangers of the keto diet.

5. Loss of Muscle Mass

You will be surprised to know that in a keto diet you will not only lose your fats but the proteins with it. This means that the weight you are losing may not only me the fats but also your muscle mass. It happens when you will not maintain the level of proteins in your diet. Your body will start burning the muscles to generate energy and, in this way, the lean muscle mass in your body will be reduced. To prevent the loss of muscle mass, you should maintain the proteins in your diet.

6. Weight Regain

Do not forget that you are eating fats for losing fats.

There are chances that you will start gaining weight instead of losing it. The reason is that there are many people who start the keto diet but their body does not enter the ketosis. This is the reason they will immediately start gaining weight instead of losing it. This is a very dangerous condition because you can turn into an obese person in no time. The best solution is to monitor the level of ketones present on your blood. It will help you know whether your body is in ketosis state or not.

7. Low Blood Sugar Level

No doubt keto diet is going for the people suffering from diabetes who have a higher blood sugar level. However, for a normal individual it can be side effects. The reason is that your body will not be able to maintain the normal level of sugar in blood because you are not consuming the carbs. This is the reason sugar level will drop below the normal limits and you will have to deal with the side effects that comes with it.

8. Dehydration

The common dangers of the keto diet is dehydration. There are chances that you are drinking the normal amount of water. However, your body will need more water to get rid of the stored ketones and other waste products that are produced by the keto diet. This is the reason your kidney will be consuming more water to flush out the wastes. In this way you may have to suffer from severe dehydration. The better solution is to assure that you consume double amount of water just like your kidney is consuming it. That is the only way you can protect yourself from dehydration and formation of kidney stones.

9. Cardiac Problems

No doubt that keto diet can help you control the level of LDL in your body. however, if you will not monitor your consumption of fats and you will keep consuming all the unhealthy fatty products, chances are you will increase the risk of heart problems. The level of LDL will increase in your body that will cause the obstruction of blood vessels. You may have to deal with various health issues like hypertension. If you will not monitor your condition properly, it may lead to various other health issues.

10. Constipation

Many people suffer from constipation after consuming the keto diet. The reason is that they do not drink enough water that can be used to pass out the stool, as well as their body is not comfortable with the fatty food items. It is taking more time for their body to digest the food items and this is the reason they are dealing with constipation. It is not minor dangers of the keto diet because constipation can lead to various other health issues. Your body is not eliminating the waste products that you have consumed, and it can lead to toxicity of the body.

CHAPTER 9

BENEFITS OF KETOGENIC

One of the hottest approaches in weight loss that is sweeping the industry is the idea of ketogenic diet weight loss programs. These are extreme low-carb diets where the aim is to be in a state of ketosis, meaning that the body is burning fat as fuel as opposed to glucose. This state is achieved, largely, by simply depriving the body of glucose via the food source is available through the dieters nutritional plan.

This is a diet approach that works for many people, and here are 5 benefits of ketogenic diets that you may not be aware of.

1. Being in ketosis allows the body to process fat and use it as fuel in a way that no other state allows as easily. Carbohydrates are much easier to convert and use as fuel, so when you are providing plenty of these to your body, you need to burn and use all of those before your body will finally begin converting and

using fat as fuel!

2. Another benefit of being in a state of ketosis is that excess ketones are not harmful to your system in any way whatsoever. Any key tones that you create which are not needed by your body are simply excreted through urine, easily and harmlessly. In fact, this excellent benefit is the reason why you can check whether you are in a state of ketosis using urine testing strips in the morning.

3. When your body gets used to being in ketosis, it will actually begin to prefer ketones to glucose. This is the ideal state that you want your body to be in - no longer craving sugar whatsoever, and in fact preferring protein as a fuel source as opposed to sugar.

4. Another benefit of ketogenic diet weight loss is that being in a ketogenic state is very useful for controlling insulin levels in the body. Insulin is one of the substances that makes you crave food, particularly for its high in sugar, and so controlling it to healthy levels is one of the key elements of weight loss.

5. Last, but certainly not least, is that the majority of people who take advantage of ketogenic diet weight loss report that being in a ketogenic state makes them feel significantly less hungry than when they are in a non-

ketogenic state. It is much easier to stick to a diet - any diet - when you're not fighting cravings and hunger every step of the way. In fact, hunger pangs can often be the thing that derails a person's best efforts! Not having to deal with them makes it easier to meet your goals, all the way around.

Now that you are aware of all of the weight loss benefits of being in a state of ketosis, it makes sense that you would at least give this approach a try - after all, what do you have to lose except weight?

With the combination of weight loss from the reduction in carbohydrates, the traditional dietary source for energy, ketonics are seen as a way to offset disease brought on by carbohydrate ingestion. Studies are showing a reduction in carbs can help control and. manage epileptic seizures, as well as a plethora of weight related diagnosis such as type 2 diabetes, obesity issues, and cardiovascular concerns related to cholesterol levels and triglyceride imbalances. Researchers are also looking toward the brain to answer questions on what is ketogenic effects on brain function, due to relations found in fats with brain tissue. It is here where epileptic management is believed to occur. Diseases such as Parkinson's,

Alzheimer's, narcolepsy, and amyotrophic lateral sclerosis are being looked at for reductions in relation to ketogenic treatments.

This is arguably the most common "intentional" use of the ketogenic diet today. It has found a niche for itself in the mainstream dieting trend. Keto diets have become part of many dieting regimen due to its well acknowledged side effect of aiding weight loss.

Though initially maligned by many, the growing number of favorable weight loss results has helped the ketogenic to better embraced as a major weight loss program.

Besides the medical benefits, ketogenic diets also provide some general health benefits which include the following

Improved Insulin Sensitivity: This is obviously the first aim of a ketogenic diet. It helps to stabilize your insulin levels thereby improving fat burning.

Muscle Preservation: Since protein is oxidized, it helps to preserve lean muscle. Losing lean muscle mass causes an individual's metabolism to slow down as muscles are generally very metabolic. Using a keto diet actually helps to preserve your muscles while your body burns fat.

Controlled pH and respiratory function: A keto diet helps to decrease lactate thereby improving both pH and respiratory function. A state of ketosis therefore helps to keep your blood pH at a healthy level.

Improved Immune System: Using a ketogenic diet helps to fight off aging antioxidants while also reducing inflammation of the gut thereby making your immune system stronger.

Reduced Cholesterol Levels: Consuming fewer carbohydrates while you are on the keto diet will help to reduce blood cholesterol levels. This is due to the increased state of lipolysis. This leads to a reduction in LDL cholesterol levels and an increase in HDL cholesterol levels.

Reduced Appetite and Cravings: Adopting a ketogenic diet helps you to reduce both your appetite and cravings for calorie rich foods. As you begin eating healthy, satisfying, and beneficial high-fat foods, your hunger feelings will naturally start decreasing.

CHAPTER 10

KETOGENIC DIET MENU PLAN FOR BEGINNERS: UNDERSTANDING SKD, TKD AND CKD

If you have decided to lose weight this spring, then you might want to consider the Ketogenic diet. The diet has been around for a long time and was once used to treat patients with epileptic or seizure problems, especially among young kids. Nowadays, the diet has lost its popularity with the advent of prescription drugs that treat the health problem. The diet however is used by many dieters around the world because of its efficacy and although diets have its side effects, knowing about the diet and following the rules can help one lose weight without compromising their overall health.

Beginners especially should have a brief overview of the diet and the meal plan to help them make an informed decision should they decide to do the diet on their own. As always, those with health problems should consult their medical health provider so that they can help patients to adjust to the meal plan or to monitor them to ensure that the ketogenic therapy will not affect their health.

TYPES OF KETOGENIC DIETS

Ketogenic diet is a high fat low carbohydrate diet with adequate protein thrown in the meal. It is further divided into three types and depending on one's daily calorie needs, the percentage differs. Diets are often prepared on a ratio level such as 4:1 or 2:1 with the first number indicating the total fat amount in the diet compared to the protein and carbohydrate combined in each meal.

Standard - SKD

The first diet is the Standard or the SKD and is designed for individuals who are not active or lead a sedentary lifestyle. The meal plan limits the dieter to eat a net of 20-50 grams of carbohydrates. Fruits or vegetables that are starchy are restricted from the diet. In order for the diet to be effective, one must strictly follow the meal plan. Butter, vegetable oil and heavy creams are used heavily to replace carbohydrates in the diet.

Targeted - TKD

The TKD is less strict than the SKD and allows one to consume carbohydrates though only in a certain portion or amount which will not impact the ketosis that one is currently in. The TKD diet helps dieters that perform some level of exercise or workout.

Cyclical - CKD

The CKD is preferable for those who are into weight training or do intensive exercises and not for beginners as it requires the person undergoing the diet to stick to a SKD meal plan for the five days in a week's time and eating/loading up on carbohydrates on the next two days. It is important that dieters follow the strict regimen to ensure that their diet is successful.

CHAPTER 11

WHAT IS THE CYCLICAL
KETOGENIC DIET?

A cyclical ketogenic diet is a plan when one follows the normal ketogenic diet from Monday to Friday along with three days of workouts. The weekend food is loaded with carbs without exercise. This stores some carbohydrate energy for the week ahead and helps to maintain a level of strength. The reason for 1 or 2 days of high carb diet is to fill the muscle energy tank. The diet is cyclic which means it is to be repeated. The weekend involves eating of foods one is craving for like bread, pizzas, and pastas. The cyclical ketogenic diet has to follow certain discipline, calculations and watching the intake of calories. The calculations vary according to the individual's age, work, gender and physical health.

The dietician advices. and induction phase of about 14 days. In this the low carb and high fat diet is given for five days and then a high fat and low carb diet fir two days. This cycle is repeated every week.The basic purpose of cyclical ketogenic diet is to lose extra fat by eating more of fat and protein. One aims to have a diet that contains 60% fat, 35% protein and 5% carbohydrates. The best form of low ketogenic diet is called cyclical ketogenic diet.

The diet breaks the protein carbs and fats into macros that help to distribute how many grams of each type of food is required daily on the low carb phase. The cyclical ketogenic diet is a diet that is a perfect low carb ketogenic diet. The low carb diet estimates the calorie count by breaking down the amount of protein, fat and carbohydrates. The best breakdown for calories from protein, carbs and fat is a 65% fat, 30% protein, 5% carbohydrates ratio. The reason the diet is called a cyclical ketogenic diet is because we spend 5 days of the week doing a low carb phase and then the next two days is a high carb, or carb up, phase.

How is Cyclical Ketogenic Diet Calculated?

The low carb food of the cyclical ketogenic diet is same to that of the standard ketogenic diet.

18 calories per pound of body weight is required for gaining mass

12 calories per pound of body weight is required to lose weight

15-16 calories per pound of body weight is required to maintain weight.

Carbohydrates have to be up to 30g per day.

Fats fill in the remainder of caloric needs.

This diet plan is a unique diet chart that includes lots of nutrients and diets. Each and every human being has his own taste and a diet should be made keeping in mind that it doesn't affect the taste. One should think of meals that have less oil and fat in them and that which are very simple to make.

If you are working, you need to carry your own tiffin. Make meals, that are very easy to carry and that which are good for your health too. One should always watch his own net carbs that should not exceed. 50-60 grams a day. This will make you feel fit. In order to avoid glycogen in your meals, you should include carbs 20-30 grams each day.

If you want to intake potassium intake in your diet, eat lite salt. To strengthen your bones in sodium have the broth of the chicken bones. But never have dairy products in your keto diet plan. Also avoid sweets that are low in carbs. If you have them you might be affected with random loss of weight. If you want to have your usual tea and coffee, use coconut milk instead of milk.

WHAT TO AVOID?

In Ketogenic diet menu plan you need to avoid certain food items:

Sugar items, syrups of corn- Avoid fruit juices, ice cream, chocolate, soft drinks, pastry, table sugar and all items that have extra sugar in them.

All grains- Avoid soft breads, loafs, pasta, wheat, barley, rye.

Dairy products- All the dairy products should be avoided.

Legumes- Avoid lentils, vegetables like beans.

Vegetable oils- All vegetable oils such as sunflower oil, olive oil, corn oil, and soyabean oil should be avoided.

Hydrogenated oils- These oils are found in margarines and other fat products and should be avoided too.

Sweeteners that are artificial: Avoid using artificial sweeteners such as Aspartame, Sucralosse, Saccharin, etc.

What to Eat? Keto Sea foods In this chart, things that you should include are as follows:

Meats, eggs, vegetables- Include chicken, mutton, beef, pork, lamb, turkey as meats. Have omega 3 rich eggs, vegetables such as onions, tomatoes, broccolis should be included too.

Seafood, fish- include good fish and seafood in your Ketogenic diet menu plan.

Fruits and Tubers- Include fruits such as apples, bananas, strawberries as fruits and also turnips and sweet potatoes as tubes.

Salts, spices- Spices and salts such as turmeric, sea salt, and garlic should be included.

Also include nuts, berries, and healthy oils in your diet charts.

CHAPTER 12

THE KETOGENIC DIET MENU PLAN MADE HERE GIVES YOU A 7 DAY DIET CHART PLAN:

THE DIET CHART

Day 1

Breakfast: Fry 2 eggs and also includes boiled vegetables, all done in coconut oil. Have an apple or any fruit you like.

Lunch: Have some nuts. Have Chicken salad done in olive oil.

Dinner: If you like Burgers, fry two in butter and have few boiled vegetables. You can have salsa too.

Day 2

Breakfast: Have a fruit. Have eggs and also bacon.

Lunch: If you like burger, fry in butter and have boiled vegetables. Have a fruit salad.

Dinner: Have salmon which you should fry in butter. Have Vegetable salad.

Day 3

Wednesday

Breakfast: Boiled vegetables with chicken or any meat you like.

Lunch: In a lettuce leaf put a sandwich; have boiled chicken and vegetable salad.

Dinner: Have Berries or nuts, beef fry, boiled vegetables.

Day 4

Breakfast: Have fried eggs and a fruit.

Lunch: Have few nuts, boiled chicken and a salad.

Dinner: Have boiled Vegetables and chicken or pork.

Day 5

Breakfast: One should have eggs and green vegetables that are fried in coconut oil.

Lunch: Have some nuts. Then also have chicken salad that is fried in olive oil.

Dinner: Have beef steak with green vegetables and include sweet potato too.

Day 6

Breakfast: Have a fruit. Have eggs and include bacon too.

Lunch: If you have leftover beef steak of the day before, have it with boiled vegetables.

Dinner: Bake a salmon in olive oil. Include avocado and some vegetables too.

Day 7

If you are thinking that Ketogenic diet menu plan will not allow you to diet in Sundays, you are wrong. You can have more meal but you have to diet every single day.

Breakfast: Have boiled vegetables and meat.

Lunch: Have a sandwich, boiled chicken and

vegetable salad in your diet.

Dinner: Grill some chicken wings in olive oil and have it with boiled vegetables and salsa.

Your ketogenic diet menu plan also includes your restaurant meals. That doesn't mean you will eat less. But eat intelligently so that your colleagues don't even understand that you are dieting. For the main dish order a fish or meat. Avoid bread or having rice and instead order more vegetables and salad. Ask the cook or the chef to cook your food in olive oil or in coconut oil.

Having Snacks

Well, apart from following this diet chat, you need to have some snacks every two hours that will help your system run properly. For the snacks, include nuts and berries, baby carrots, boiled eggs, a fruit, slices of apple fried in almond butter, beef steak made at home, any leftovers of previous night. All these will enhance the positive levels in your Ketogenic diet menu plan.

Apart from all these you can have tea and coffee since tea has antioxidants. You can include green tea which is good for your health. You can also search on internet best Ketogenic diet menu plan recipes that are easy and very quick to make. Make them at home and serve yourself. You will feel great!

We have been told our entire life that the primary source of energy for our body is sugar. However, there are many other efficient sources of energy that can be utilized by our body and one of them is ketones. Ketones are produced when fats are metabolized by our body and these ketones are used by the cells as a source of energy for their normal functions. Ketosis is a metabolic state in which the level of ketones is increased in the body. In order to achieve ketosis, the normal level of ketones in the blood should be 0.5 mmol/L. In order to achieve ketosis, you have to consume Ketosis diet that is high in fats with adequate proteins and lower carbs. It will help your body to go into ketosis.

Experts are continuously working on the Ketosis diet to reveal many benefits that come with the system. There are many people who are planning to start a Ketosis diet because they want to achieve better mental performance, manage their weight and prevent their body from various diseases. However, the real issue is that they do not have a complete understanding of ketosis and ketosis diet. They want to know whether this new approach would be beneficial for them or not. Here we have a complete guideline that will answer your questions and resolve all your doubts related to the Ketosis diet.

When approaching a new diet, it might be a good time to reflect what is ketogenic? As with many dietary considerations, the focus comes down to carbohydrates, though not all low-carb diets can be considered ketonic in nature. Many plans, such as the Atkins, start with a drastic reduction in carbs, but will gradually increase them to maintain the plan's balance. What begins as ketogenic eventually dissipates and becomes something else. Knowing what is ketogenic conditioning will help maintain your plan for a diet's end result, and help maintain the effects long after you have started. Ketosis, the basis for any ketogenic diet, is a state the body enters where it is not receiving the glucose required for energy, so it moves into a state where ketone molecules become generated during the metabolism of fats. These ketones are then used as supplemental energy sources.

CHAPTER 13

<u>LOW CARB FOODS THAT YOU'VE GOT TO INCLUDE IN YOUR MENU</u>

There are many people who are planning to start the keto diet. They have planned everything from the healthy fatty ingredients that they are going to use in their diet to how they are planning to maintain the level of proteins in their body. They have even prepared their list of ingredients and all other items that they need to assure that they will not have to deal with any issues while following the keto diet. However, a common issue that people have to deal with while following the keto diet is that they get bored with the food they are consuming. There are many people who complain that the food is not very interesting and flavorful. This is the reason they are unable to maintain the diet plan. In order to deal with this issue, they have to add flavors to their meal and they do not know how to make it possible.

Want to enjoy a slim and lean frame? Well, in that case, you've got to include some viable and necessary low carbohydrate diet foods. These diet foods will not only make you lean but they'll also buck up your muscle strength and help you enjoy a perfect and strong frame. Now, in case you're perplexed with the innumerable low carb foods to pick from, we've sorted an easy list for you. This list comes with every necessary low carb food that is good for your body. Take a look.

LOW CARB FOOD LIST

Meats

For meats, you can choose from chicken breast, turkey, pork, lean ground beef, and lean cuts of steak, lamb, veal and even ham. Following is a list of top two meats that you've got to have for a slimmer and slender frame right away.

Chicken breast

Chicken breast is one of the most essential low carb foods that have to be in your diet list. This food not only has high protein content, but it is also low in fat and extra calories. To add to the benefits, you can cook chicken breast in any possible variation.

Ground Turkey

If you are looking for food which is low in carbohydrates and fats, but extremely high in proteins, Ground Turkey can be a great option. Ground Turkey can be cooked up with almost anything and seasoned with a dash of savory spices for taste. This meat will never disappoint you.

Fishes and seafood

Among fishes, Salmon, Tuna, Tilapia, cod and shrimps should definitely make their place in your diet.

Tuna

Wild caught Tuna is great for your body as it comes loaded with omega 3 fatty acids. However, always try to go for the wild caught variants of Tuna instead of the canned ones.

Salmon

Salmon is one of those protein foods that are extremely low in carbs. In fact, salmon has more of omega 3 fatty acids and protein. Salmon can be a perfect food in your low fat diet plan for its versatility and health benefits.

Nuts and seeds

Nuts and grains like almond, Cashew, pistachio,

walnuts, pumpkin seeds, sunflower seeds and flax seeds are extremely necessary for your low carb diet.

Cashew

Cashew is loaded with good fats, omega 3 fatty acids and lots of protein. The fiber content of this nut is also pretty commendable. So, if you're making a diet list minus the carbs, cashew can always make its place in the list.

Pumpkin Seeds

Pumpkin seeds are extremely necessary to make any and every meal delectable. Apart from being delectable, they are also very healthy and nutritious. The high protein content in these adds to the benefits.

Other foods

Other common foods like peanut butter, tofu, edmame, chickpeas, black beans and even hummus are great for your diet. These foods are low in carbohydrates and rich in protein and healhy fats.

So, simply go through the list of necessary diet foods and follow this regime for a slim, slender and flab free body in the long run.

LOW CARB DIET RECIPE

When following a keto diet, people cannot add bread into their daily diet. That's because bread has the ability to provide carbs to the body. Hence, the consumption of bread has the ability to keep people away from achieving the state of ketosis. But still, they will be able to go ahead and enjoy keto bread. Keto bread might not be available in your local bakery to purchase. But you don't need to worry about anything because you can simply prepare keto bread at the comfort of your own home. Below mentioned are the steps that you will have to follow when you are preparing keto bread at your home.

CHAPTER 14

<u>INGREDIENTS REQUIRED</u>
<u>FOR KETO BREAD</u>

As the first thing of preparing this recipe, it is important to understand what ingredients are needed. When all the ingredients are there by your side, you can simply proceed with the preparation of the recipe.

- 3 egg whites
- One cup of boiling water
- 2 teaspoons of apple cider vinegar
- 1 teaspoon of sea salt
- 2 teaspoons of baking powder
- 5 teaspoons of husk powder
- 1 cup of almond flour
- 2 tablespoons of sesame seeds

All these ingredients can be purchased from your

local grocery store. You don't have to spend a fortune on these as well. It is important to keep in mind that the last ingredient in the recipe, sesame seeds are optional. If you want to enhance the flavor of keto bread, you can go for it. Otherwise, you can stick to the other ingredients that are mentioned in this recipe.

Steps to Follow

Once all ingredients are available on your kitchen countertop, you can simply proceed with the below mentioned steps and prepare keto bread.

As the first thing, you will need to pre heat your oven. It is recommended for you to pre heat the oven for a temperature of 350 degrees Fahrenheit. While your oven is heating up, you can simply mix all the dry ingredients that you have inside a large bowl. Then you will be able to reduce the time taken to prepare this recipe.

As the next step, you will have to boil water and add into your mixture. Along with water, you should add egg whites and vinegar as well. Then you can start beating the mixture. It is recommended for you to grab a hand mixture and beat it for a period of 30 seconds. You need to be careful not to over mix your dough. If you do, you will not be able to end up with the best tasting keto bread.

Once mixing is completed, you can simply moisten

your hands and prepare six different pieces of dough. Then you can take a baking sheet, and apply grease on it. The pieces of dough should then be placed on top of the baking sheet.

Now you need to insert dough into the oven. You are encouraged to bake it for a period of about 60 minutes in a lower rack. But if the space is not enough, you can use another rack inside the oven. Once you start hearing the hollow sound of bun tapping the bottom, you need to figure out that bread has been baked perfectly. Hence, you need to take it out and prepare for serving.

After taking keto bread out from the oven, you can keep it for few minutes to cool down. It is recommended for you to serve this along with butter. Or else, you are provided with the freedom to choose any other topping based on your preferences.

The best thing about keto bread is that it doesn't contain any carbs. Hence, you will be provided with the ability to remain within the state of ketosis. You can even consume keto bread on a daily basis. If you can do it, your body will tend to use fat deposited in different areas of the body as energy. Hence, you will be able to burn fat in an efficient manner. Fat burning means that you will be provided with the ability to reduce your weight. Hence, you will absolutely love to consume the keto bread recipe.

THE KETOGENIC MUFFINS

The ketogenic muffin is a delight to the taste buds and it is a storehouse of the necessary nutrients of to keep healthy. These muffins are the preparation that comes in the category of the ketogenic diet. Hence, the recipe ensures the balanced supply of protein-fiber-fats and carbohydrates.

A Breakfast Recipe That Combines Health and Delicacies

The hectic schedule of life seldom offers you the time that you can put to prepare a lavish breakfast. However, you cannot ignore the perspectives of health benefits and of course you have to show some care for your taste buds as well. The ketogenic muffin is a recipe proposed that you can prepare fast and would comes delicious as well as beneficial from the point of nutrition. The preparation involves the following ingredients:

- Golden Flaxseed: 25 O
- Coca powder: 5 Oz
- Cinnamon: 1 tablespoon
- Baking powder: ½ tablespoon
- Salt: ½ tea spoon
- Coconut oil: 25 ML

- Caramel syrup: 50 ml

- Vanilla extract: 10 ml

- Apple-cider vinegar: 5 ml

- Silvered Almonds: 4/5 Oz

The Steps to Prepare

1. You require pre-heating the oven to a temperature of 350 degree F

2. Take all the dry ingredients into a mixing bowl and go on stirring till it mixes well

3. In a separate bowl, mix all the wet ingredients together

4. Combine the dry and wet ingredients

5. Take the mixture into muffin liners.

6. You require sprinkling the silver almonds as the toppings on each muffin

7. Bake the batter for about 15 minutes. The ketogenic muffin has to swell up to come to the top

8. Serve

ABOUT THE NUTRITIONAL CONTENT

The ketogenic muffin would offer you 12 grams of protein, 10 grams of fibers, 14 grams of fats and 4 grams of carbohydrates over each of its servings. Hence, approach the preparation to get rewarded dually with impeccable taste and the highest nutritional benefits.

Why Should You Opt For The Ketogenic Muffins?

The ketogenic muffin is a store house for the nutritional values. Each of the serving is loaded with the perfect balance of high protein & fat and the minimal of carbohydrate. Note that the fat that the muffins contain gets converted to energy instantly and hence, it would energize you but would never trigger obesity.

It is advised to refrain from the ketogenic muffin in case you are suffering from high cholesterol related troubles.

CREAMY KETO QUESADILLAS

Creamy keto quesadillas is the best products available in the market. It is filled with creamy deliciousness that would be hard for you to ignore. Ingredients

- 2 tbsp Coconut flour
- 2 tbsp Heavy cream
- 1 Egg
- 1 tbsp Olive oil (for cooking)
- 2 oz Mushrooms
- 1 oz Spinach
- 1 oz Cream cheese
- 4 tbsp Parmesan cheese

Instructions

1. Take a mixing bowl and add coconut flour and egg in it. Mix it properly to assure that it is smooth.

2. In the tortilla mixture you have to add some heavy cream and mix it properly until it is smooth

3. Take a pan and it keep it on medium heat. Add olive oil to the main and wait until it is hot. You have to pour the mixture into the pan and

cook it properly into a tortilla.

4. You have to cook your tortilla just like a pan cake from both sides.

5. Take another sauce pain and melt your parmesan and cream cheese in it.

6. Add spinach and mushrooms into the melted cheese and sauté it properly.

7. Once the mixture is prepared and cooked properly you have to add it onto your tortillas that you have prepared previously. Fold on one side and enjoy your perfect meal.

FRIED BACON AND EGGS

People who prepare their meals by following keto diet experience major improvements to their health and weight loss. However, eating nothing but low-carb, high-fat foods can get repetitive after a while. If you like to eat bacon and eggs in the morning, but are getting tired of preparing them the same way, this article will help you expand your collection of ketogenic breakfast recipes with a delicious new entry. The following recipe for bacon and eggs brings out the unique flavors of both ingredients, while also retaining their nutritional value, and the addition of carrots and onions fits them surprisingly well.

As with most other ketogenic breakfast recipes, it's simple enough for you to add some more variety to the process once you've gotten familiar with it. It's also so easy to prepare and clean up that you'll often find yourself wanting to fry some bacon and eggs in the middle of the day, not just in the morning. If you need more options for your ketogenic breakfast, you can take a look spinach omelet with white eggs recipe here. For much more recipes for breakfast, visit our ketogenic breakfast recipes category.

The Ingredients Include:

- Butter (1 tablespoon)

- Bacon (8 slices)

- One carrot (peeled).

- Broccoli (chopped, ½ cup)

- Celery (chopped, ½ cup)

- One half of a large white onion (chopped)

- Four large eggs

- Cheese (shredded, ½ cup)

Instructions

1. Slice pieces of meaty bacon into smaller strips across the grain.

2. Belt 1 tablespoon of butter in a large frying pan over medium heat.

3. Put the peeled carrot, broccoli and celery inside the pan to sauté in the butter for about 20 minutes, until the vegetables start to caramelize and bacon becomes crisp around the edges. Remember to stir frequently.

4. Spread everything evenly on the frying pan.

5. Free some room in each quarter section for eggs. Break an egg into each resulting space.

6. Keep cooking until the eggs are nearly done. If you prefer cooked yolks, put the lid over the frying pan and wait for the eggs to cook through in steam.

7. Otherwise, just let the whites cook and turn the eggs over to leave the yolk mostly liquid.

8. Once the eggs are nearly ready, spread the shredded cheese evenly on top and leave it until it melts. You can turn the heat off or leave it for a while longer depending on your preference.

9. Finally, serve the hot meal and enjoy a delicious new entry to your collection of healthy ketogenic breakfast recipes.

NOTES

Even though they contain a significant amount of carbohydrates, vegetables are essential to most ketogenic breakfast recipes. Broccoli is one of the best choices because it's relatively low-carb when compared to most other vegetables, but it can also be replaced with cauliflower or some other type of green leafy vegetables.

Carrots and celery can also be replaced with a similar amount of turnips. Cut them up and cook them together with onions, long enough to see them caramelize. The result will be just as delicious and add some much needed variety to your breakfast table and the rest of ketogenic breakfast recipes.

HIGH PROTEIN KETO CHICKEN QUESADILLAS

In case you think your diet is getting low on proteins you can enjoy this high protein keto quesadillas. Here is the complete recipe that you have to follow.

Ingredients

- 4 Crepes or you can prepare your own at home
- 1 cup Chicken breast (cooked and diced)
- ½ cup Sweet pepper diced
- ¼ cup Red onions diced
- 2 cups Mozzarella cheese
- 1 tbsp Avocado oil

Instructions

1. Take a cast iron skillet and keep it over a medium heat. Add avocado oil to heat it properly.

2. In the heated oil you have to add your chicken and fry it properly. Once it is fried you can add your veggies. Keep them crunchy or soft the way that you like.

3. Evenly cook your meal and add your favorite dressing into the pan to add more flavor to the

meal.

4. Take a large bowl and transfer all your ingredients into it

5. Take another bowl and add cheese and dressings to it. Mix it properly until it is smooth and cheese is evenly coated.

6. Take another non-stick pan and spray a little oil on it. Cook your tortillas properly on the pan

7. Once the tortillas are cooked you have to set them on a plate. Spread the cheese properly and add the mixture of chicken and veggies to the mixture. After that add more cheese.

8. Fold your tortilla in half and pat with the spatula to assure that it is set properly.

9. Serve while it is hot with your favorite keto drink.

LOW CARB PIZZA RECIPE

If you are currently on a low carb diet, like the ketogenic diet, but suddenly feel like eating a slice of pizza, there is nothing better than a homemade pizza recipe. This low carb pizza recipe is packed with nutritious and delicious ingredients that will surely give you an energy boost. Everyone should give the low carb pizza a try, even if only once.

Ingredients

This is a low carb pizza recipe that uses bacon too, because everyone loves bacon. These are the ingredients: 1 or 2 tbs coconut oil, 1 big cauliflower head, 1 large onion, 1 tbs margarine, some water, 2 eggs, 2 teaspoons of your favorite seasoning, 2 cups of shredded mozzarella cheese, some shredded parmesan, half pound bacon, 1 jar of Ragu pizza sauce, and a blend of 5 of your favorite cheese types. Read the labels to choose the ones with lowest carb content. The lower carb content, the better for your low carb pizza. And, you will learn how to prepare your pizza, calories, nutritional values and more right now. If you need more recipes for your ketogenic diet, you can take a look our ketogenic diet recipes category.

HOW TO PREPARE YOUR PIZZA

The crust of the low carb pizza is the most complicated one to make. You need to preheat the oven and prepare a 17 by 11 cookie sheet, if it fits in your oven. Saute the chopped cauliflower with the chopped onion, in butter, in a large skillet. Add the water and make sure the. cauliflower got soft, at which point you transfer to a bowl to chill. It's time to cook the bacon. Use the food processor to puree the cauliflower, and then scrape it onto another bowl. It's time to mix it with the eggs, mozzarella, parmesan, spices, and then to spread the mixture onto the cookie sheet. Now you can see your low carb pizza starting to come together.

The crust of the low carb pizza must be baked for some 20 minutes, until it is brown on the edges. Get a sauce pan, drop the Ragu in it, the bacon broken into smaller pieces, and bring to a slow simmer. Change the oven's setting to broiling. It is time to spread the sauce on the crust, then with the cheese mixture, and put the pizza back in the oven until the cheese melts, and become brown. Now your low carb pizza should be done. Cut it into 12 pieces, and serve. Also if you need to learn a ketogenic diet menu you can find more information from our categories!

One slice of this low carb pizza should have about

315 calories, 20 grams of fat, 8 grams of carbs, 1 gram of fiber, and 21 grams of protein.

Of course, you can substitute some of the ingredients, such as using mushrooms and peppers instead of bacon. You can even use olives on top of the pizza. If you think 5 types of cheese is too much on a single pizza, use less. Doing this will alter the nutritional quantities as well. You can give up the onion if you don't like it, or use broccoli instead of cauliflower, for a more colorful, unique looking low carb pizza. Just make sure those who you want to share the low carb pizza with, also enjoy vegetables.

The keto pancake is an extremely tasty and healthy stuff that supplies the perfect blending of the protein-fat-carbohydrate with the bonus of pampering the taste buds impeccably. These pancakes would be the perfect recipe to adapt to the ketonic diet.

Ingredients

Keto pancake is a yummy delicacy that balances the perspectives of healthy and tasty foods in the equilibrium. The preparation involves the following ingredients:

- Protein powder: 6 OZ

- Sugar: 8 OZ

- Butter: 2 cubes

- Coconut Oil: 35 ML

- Almond Milk: 50 ML

- Egg: 1 (large)

- Salt: as per taste

- Caramel Syrup: 5 ML

- Baking powder: 1 teaspoon

- Coconut Floor: 8 OZ

- Vanilla essence: ½ teaspoon

Preparation

1. The recipe to prepare the keto pancake can be listed as follows:

2. Mix the flour, baking powder, sugar and salt in a large size bowl

3. In the centre of the mixture, make a well like structure and pour egg yolk, protein powder, almond milk, vanilla essence and Carmel syrup into the well.

4. Keep stirring the mixture till it blends well

5. Heat the frying pan in medium temperature. Pour the coconut oil into the pan

6. Pour the mixture into the hot oil and spread the dough evenly

7. Let the keto pancake swell up

8. Remove from the oven and garnish with butter cubes

9. Serve

POINTS TO REMEMBER WHILE PREPARING THE PANCAKES

While preparing the keto pancake, you should refrain from over mixing the dough. Likewise, it would be better to use the softened butter than the butter in molten state. You should void pressing and ideally cook less.

Is the Pancake Only to Serve The Taste Buds?

The keto pancake assembles the dimensions like fine recipes and high food values. The pan cake would be loaded with high protein and would have the minimal of carbohydrate. Hence, it can be said the delightful taste is just the bonus on high nutritional benefits.

The biggest benefit in consuming the keto pancake is that you get the perfect blending of high protein-higher counts of fats and the minimal carbohydrate that makes the preparation the perfect recipe for the ketonic diet.

If you are wondering what's the big secret of losing weight and staying healthy and fit, then the answer probably would be a strong and healthy breakfast. But, what a strong and healthy breakfast means? For most nutrition and diet specialists it means 60% carbs, 25% protein and 15% fats. Following this scheme, the meal that best suits it is egg white spinach omelet. And here's why.

Egg White Spinach Omelet and Nutritional Values

Firstly, eggs is the crucial protein container for everyday menu. One egg (whole) contains 96 calories, of which 11% of fat (7.3 g), 10% of saturated fat (2g), 64% of cholesterol (191mg), 4% of sodium (98mg), and 6.5g of proteins. One egg also. contains 3% calcium and 5% iron, so it's a valuable source of these minerals too. Don't be scared of confused with high level of cholesterol, because it won't hurt your overall cholesterol level if you eat eggs twice a week.

On the other hand, spinach is a great ingredient in everyone's daily menu because of its low calorie value (15 calories for a cup of spinach), and its high level of iron and calcium. As you may know, green leafy vegetables are desirable in every nutrition plan because the level of calcium and iron is at highest in them. So, basically, you have a lot of healthy things in just 100 calories!

One of the most popular recipes for egg white spinach omelet goes as follows:

- Egg whites (4–5)
- Egg yolks (1)
- Almond milk (30 ml)

- Tomato (one half)

- Shredded spinach (1 handful)

- Purple Onion (1 tabs)

- Basil (1 pence)

- Olive oil cooking spray

- Garlic (optional)

HOW TO PREPARE YOUR MEAL

First, chop the veggies (tomato and onion) in one bowl and beat egg whites, egg yolk and almond milk in the other. Spray a small frying pan with olive oil and just quick sauté the veggies (only to soften them). When finished, put veggies on the side, spray the pan again, put medium-low heat, and pour the eggs. Once the eggs got firm, put the veggies on one side, and fold the other half over the top. You can serve it with fresh fruits, to boost your metabolism even more!

The choice of fruits is yours, but you should probably use some with lots of fibers, or some citrus fruits. Egg white spinach omelet prepared in this way contains 203 calories (just omelet, without fruits!). 5g of fat, 20 g of proteins and 18 g of carbs make this dish suitable for breakfast, lunch, or dinner. It also contains 272 mg of sodium, 8g of sugar, and 2g of fiber. So, it's a little nutrition bomb, especially for those who lacks energy in the morning and who needs to follow a strict, low-carb/high-protein diet plan with exhausting physical training.

A great tip: you can prepare this egg white spinach omelet in advance, pack it in a lunch box and put it in a wrap (either gluten free or whole grain) for a healthy meal on the go. Or, you can just eat it with some lemonade on the side! Enjoy! Do you often miss bun burgers in your stringent Ketogenic diet regime? Well, in case you do, we've figured out some awesome solutions to help you out. Yep! We've listed the ideas of making 3 delectable and scrumptious ketogenic bun burger, minus the carbs and gluten. Read on, for a quick and complete insight on making these lip smacking burgers. You will definitely love the ideas.

ALMOND BUN BURGERS

Burgers are incredibly delectable, and when they come with a dash of almond they turn out to be even tastier. Here's a recipe of an awesome almond bun burger that comes with the perfect dose of taste and health. For this burger, you will need some large quantities of. almond flour, considerably large eggs, flour and un-salted butter, a dash of salt, around two tablespoons of splenda and half tablespoons of baking powder. You can use any substitute of splenda if it is not available for you.

The recipe is considerably simple compared to other complicated and tedious recipes of bun burgers. Here, you have to begin by whisking the dry ingredients in a bowl. You've got to do the whisking well enough to ensure that it is proper and viable. As soon as the ingredients are combined perfectly, you have to now add eggs to the mixture. Follow this up by dividing the mixture properly and equally in 6 parts. After that, place the stuff on a muffin pan or any equivalent equipment. Bake it for 15-20 minutes and your buns are soon ready. These buns will turn out to be downright fluffy and delectable. Add lots of veggies and bacon in between the burgers to make them delectable and scrumptious. This is probably one of the best homemade keto burgers you have ever tasted.

WHOLE WHEAT BURGER BUNS

Whole Wheat is great for your body and when you use this wheat to make burgers, they turn out to be even more delectable. Now, following is the recipe of an awesome and extremely tantalizing whole wheat burger that abides by the keto diet and comes with a burst of awesome flavors. You will need a cup of water, a cup of low fat milk, a package of dry yeast, one large egg that is in the room temperature, two teaspoons of sugar, two teaspoons of salt, a tablespoon of extra virgin oil or the cranola oil, 3/4th cups of whole wheat flour, 3/4th cups of all-purpose flour and a dash of cornmeal for sprinkling.

For these burger buns, heat milk in a medium flame for 10 minutes. While you do it, pour water in a bowl and stir it for around 5-10 minutes. Beat vigorously and try at least 100 strokes of beating. Soon add the whole wheat flour, 1/3rd cup at a time. When the dough is no longer longer sticky transfer it to a floured surface and knead it for 7-8 minutes. Now, cover the entire thing with plastic and keep it for around 1-2 hours.

When the dough will double, take it to a floured surface and knead it for around a minute or two. After this, cut it in 8 pieces (equal in size). Now, coat a huge baking sheet with proper cooking spray and dust it with cornmeal. Shape the dough in tight balls and place it on the tray. Coat a large plastic sheet with the cooking spray. Now set the buns warm until they have risen a little. Let the bun rise a little more and cook the stuff for twenty more minutes. Preheat the oven with 375 degrees and bake the buns until they are golden and crusty. So, simply try these recipes at home for an awesome burst of delectable flavors.

In an era where losing weight has become the latest trend, the majority of the population tend to be nervous about what they consume as food and beverages. Especially they feel guilty about having desserts. A misconception has been rooted in the society for decades which states that oily desserts lead to health hazards such as strokes, cholesterol and diabetes and gaining weight. On the contrary low carb high fat ketogenic desserts could eliminate above mentioned health issue while gifting you longevity. This book principal objective is to discuss benefits and nutritional values of a delicious, healthy and easy to make ketogenic dessert.

HOW TO PREPARE COCONUT CREAM MACAROONS

- 1 teaspoon vanilla
- 4 or 5 egg whites
- 1/4 teaspoon cream of tartar
- 9 ounces cream cheese
- 1 cup erythritol
- 3 ounces heavy cream
- 1/8 teaspoon salt
- 18 ounces dried coconut

To prepare this mouth watering ketogenic dessert you need to get some delicately shredded dried coconut, egg whites, cream cheese, heavy cream, cream of tartar, erythritol, vanilla, salt, unsweetened white chocolate syrup and semi sweetened chocolate chips. Once you are ready.. with the ingredients whisk egg whites, cream of tartar, vanilla and salt together. Occasionally sprinkle erythritol and whisk to the point where you could see hard peaks in the mixture. Add coconut and keep the mixture aside. Then whisk cream cheese, heavy cream and chocolate syrup together. Now mix well while adding the previous mixture. Add chocolate chips at the end. Scoop the mixture and place on a cookie sheet to bake. Bake for around 25 minutes in a 325F preheated oven. Then leave the macaroons in the oven for another 30 minutes to dry. Voila! Your scrumptious ketogenic dessert is ready to serve.

KETOGENIC DESSERT BENEFITS

The above ketogenic macaroons are made from several nutritious ketogenic foods like coconut, egg whites, cream cheese, heavy milk etc. that could force your body to enter the ketosis state to boost the fat burning process. Ketosis is the state where the body converts fat into energy instead of glycogen. This happens only if the body lack carbohydrate for the conversion. The fat to carbohydrate to protein ratio of each macaroon is 7:3:2.

This wholesome ketogenic dessert also contains 78

calories per macaroon. Beside the main advantage of increasing the number of ketones in the body which directly affect the fat burning process; ketogenic foods possess the amazing abilities of lowering the risk heart disease and Alzheimer, controlling cancers and seizure of epilepsy patients etc. There's no room for more doubts. Try out this simple recipe and share a healthy and delicious ketogenic dessert with your loved ones.

CHICKEN AND SAUSAGE KETO QUESADILLAS

Here we have one of the best keto quesadillas that you can enjoy at any moment that you like. The best thing about this keto quesadilla is that you can even prepare it for your guests and show them your amazing cooking skills.

Ingredients

- 8 Turkey sausage patties
- 1-2 tsp Olive oil
- 4 Low carb flour tortillas
- 1 1/3 cup Grated cheddar cheese
- Sause of your choice for serving

Instructions

1. Take a frying pan and heat 1 teaspoon of olive oil in it.

2. Add sausage patties into the pan over the medium heat and cook it properly. You have to assure that it is brown on both side. It will take 3 to 4 minutes to prepare the sausage.

3. Once prepared place the sausages on a cutting board and cut them in half.

4. Add a small amount of oil on the pan again and cook your tortillas properly.

5. Once the tortillas are cooked you have to sprinkle them with cheese to slightly cover the surface. After that place your sausages on the tortilla and fold them in half.

6. Keep the tortillas on the pan for a few more minutes to assure that the inside is cooked and the cheese is properly melted in the tortilla.

7. You can add your favorite dressing into the tortilla that you like and serve while it is hot.

KETO AVOCADO PIE RECIPE

Keto Avocado Pie can be considered as one of the most delicious treats available for you to enjoy. You will be able to prepare this recipe at the comfort of your own home as well. In order to do that, you just need to follow one of the keto avocado pie recipes. Below mentioned is the recipe that you will need to follow in order to prepare keto avocado pie at the comfort of your own home. Any person who is interested in preparing keto avocado pie will be able to try out this recipe. If you are on a keto diet, this would be one of the best options available for you to try out. It can help you to remain within the state of ketosis, without encountering any health issues.

INGREDIENTS REQUIRED FOR KETO AVOCADO PIE

As the first thing, you should figure out the ingredients that are required to prepare keto avocado pie. Below mentioned are the ingredients that you should find. All these ingredients can be purchased from your local stores. Hence, you will not have to worry about anything when you try out this recipe.

- Four tablespoons of coconut flour

- Four tablespoons of sesame seeds

- ¾ cup of almond flour

- One pinch of salt

- One teaspoon of baking powder

- One tablespoon of psyllium husk powder

- Four tablespoons of water

- One egg

- Three tablespoons of coconut oil or olive oil

There is a separate list of ingredients that you need in order to prepare the filling that you use for keto avocado pie. Below mentioned are the ingredients you should buy to prepare this recipe.

- One cup of mayonnaise

- Two ripe avocados

- Three eggs

- Quarter teaspoon of salt

- Half teaspoon of onion powder

- One red chili pepper

- Two tablespoons of finely chopped cilantro

- Quarter cup of shredded cheese

- Eight tablespoons of creamy cheese

Once you have all these ingredients ready, you can get started with preparing keto avocado pie recipe. Below mentioned are the instructions that you will need to follow when you are preparing the recipe.

Steps to Follow

1. As the first step, you will need to pre-heat your oven to a temperature of 350 degrees Fahrenheit. While you oven is heating up, you will need to take a food processor and mix all ingredients that you use for the pie dough. After the ingredients are mixed, you will need to wait for several minutes until it creates a ball. But if you don't have a food processor, you don't need to worry about anything because you can simply mix all ingredients inside a bowl. You can use your hands or a fork to mix these ingredients.

2. As the second step, you will have to attach a parchment paper piece to a spring form pan. It should not be longer than 12 inches in diameter. This will provide an excellent assistance for you to remove the pie after the baking process is completed.

3. Next, you need to pour dough into your pan. You can either use your fingers or an oiled spatula to get the job done. Then you can pre-bake the crust for a period of about 15

minutes.

4. As the next step, you must split avocado. You will need to remove the peel, dice and pit. In addition, you should remove seeds from avocado as well. Then you should place them inside the bowl and mix along with other ingredients.

5. Now you have come to the final step, where you will be pouring the complete mixture to the pie crust. After you pour, you must bake for a period of around 35 minutes. When you see a light golden brownish color, you should figure out that the right time has come for you to take the mixture out. Then you should let it cool for few minutes, after taking out of the oven.

KETO CHOCOLATE DONUTS

Do you always crave for chocolate donuts? Well, you don't have to order it from bakery shops every time. You can prepare them right at your home. Have you tried making it? If your answer is a boo, it is time when you should definitely do it. Chocolate is one such ingredient that is loved by everyone. In fact, donuts also have a very special place in every person's heart. They can connect donuts with several childhood memories.

Combining chocolate and donuts is a killer combo that is extremely difficult to resist. Every time you visit to a bakery shop, you always look out for the attractive and the delicious chocolate donuts. Have you ever thought that they can be prepared quite easily at your home's kitchen as well? In case you haven't ever given a try, it is the time, when you should definitely make an effort to prepare chocolate donuts. Let us find out the recipe.

The Main Ingredients

- Eggs – 3
- Ground almonds – half cup
- Baking powder – 1/4 teaspoon
- Pure cocoa powder – 2 table spoon

- Vanilla – 1 teaspoon

- Salt – 1/4 teaspoon

- Cinnamon – 1/4 teaspoon

- Melted butter – 2 tablespoon

- Splenda – half cup

- Heavy cream of almond milk – 2 tablespoon

- 100% casein protein powder of any flavour – 2 scoops

THE METHOD OF PREPARATION KETO DONUTS

1. At 350 degrees Fahrenheit preheat the oven

2. Egg whites needs to be whipped until they form hard peaks

3. Combine the splenda, egg yolks and butter in another bowl and stir it well

4. Combine all the dry ingredients and mix it well

1. Gently mix all the wet elements into the bowl of whipped egg white

2. Add the dry ingredients slowly to the bowl of wet ones and mix them well.

3. Fill the donut pan with the batter

4. Baking should be for around 15 minutes

5. Take a separate bowl and mix the heavy cream and the casein protein and stir it until it is thick.

6. Once the donuts are baked, let them rest and serve.

What Are The Add-Ons?

Add walnuts

Maple syrup can be used for dressing

Whipped heavy cream is an apt option as well.

Donuts are one such food item that is eaten across the globe and people simply love them. Several flavors are available but chocolate donuts seem to be the most popular one. You can save money when you start making restaurant quality donuts at home.

KETO PANCAKES RECIPE FOR KETOGENIC DESSERTS

The keto pancake is an extremely tasty and healthy stuff that supplies the perfect blending of the protein-fat-carbohydrate with the bonus of pampering the taste buds impeccably. These pancakes would be the perfect recipe to adapt to the ketonic diet.

Ingredients:

Keto pancake is a yummy delicacy that balances the perspectives of healthy and tasty foods in the equilibrium. The preparation involves the following ingredients:

- Protein powder: 6
- Sugar: 8 OZ
- Butter: 2 cubes

- Coconut Oil: 35 ML

- Almond Milk: 50 ML

- Egg: 1 (large)

- Salt: as per taste

- Caramel Syrup: 5 ML

- Baking powder: 1 teaspoon

- Coconut Floor: 8 OZ

- Vanilla essence: ½ teaspoon

Instruction

The recipe to prepare the keto pancake can be listed as follows:

1. Mix the flour, baking powder, sugar and salt in a large size bowl

2. In the centre of the mixture, make a well like structure and pour egg yolk, protein powder, almond milk, vanilla essence and Carmel syrup into the well.

3. Keep stirring the mixture till it blends well

4. Heat the frying pan in medium temperature. Pour the coconut oil into the pan

5. Pour the mixture into the hot oil and spread the dough evenly

6. Let the keto pancake swell up

7. Remove from the oven and garnish with butter cubes

8. Serve

Points to Remember While Preparing The Pancakes

While preparing the keto pancake, you should refrain from over mixing the dough. Likewise, it would be better to use the softened butter than the butter in molten state. You should void pressing and ideally cook less.

Is The Pancake Only to Serve The Taste Buds?

The keto pancake assembles the dimensions like fine recipes and high food values. The pan cake would be loaded with high protein and would have the minimal of carbohydrate. Hence, it can be said the delightful taste is just the bonus on high nutritional benefits.

The biggest benefit in consuming the keto pancake is that you get the perfect blending of high protein-higher counts of fats and the minimal carbohydrate that makes the preparation the perfect recipe for the ketonic diet.

CHICKEN KETO QUESADILLAS

It is one of the best and most delicious keto quesadillas that you could make at home. It has just the right amount of protein and other nutrients that will allow you to enjoy the healthy meal in the most efficient way.

Ingredients

- 3 oz Pepper jack
- 2.5 oz Chicken breast grilled
- 1/2 Avocado sliced thin
- 1 tsp Chopped jalapeño
- 1 Low carb wrap
- 1/4 tsp Dried basil
- 1/4 tsp Crushed red pepper
- 1/4 tsp Garlic powder
- 1/4 tsp Salt

Instructions

1. Grill the chicken properly o the pan. You can grill your vegetables as well if you like or you can enjoy them fresh in the quesadilla.

2. Once the chicken and vegetables are prepared,

heat the pan again to cook your tortillas on it.

3. Cook the tortillas on both sides and place the cheese on one side and cover it with chicken.

4. Wait until the cheese has melted, fold the tortilla and serve while it is hot.

CHOCOLATE KETO BROWNIES

Brownies are an all-time favorite snack. Kids and grownups love it equally. This simple recipe can be prepared right at home. Become the master of brownies. Who doesn't love chocolate brownies, and they are available in so many different types. Whenever you visit the bakery shop, you cannot resist eating one or two and also buy a few of them, right. Well, this seems to be the story of all those who have a sweet tooth. If you are looking for a weight loss regime, eating brownies can be a disaster. But can you resist the temptation? Perhaps the answer is a big no, right? Eat the brownies and do some exercise and you won't feel the guilt at all. You can prepare delicious chocolate brownies right at your home.

The Ingredients Required

- Cream cheese (6 tablespoon)
- Eggs-3
- Cocoa powder (2 tablespoon)
- Coconut oil (3 tablespoon)
- Coconut flour (1/4teaspoon)
- Almond flour (1/4 teaspoon)
- Vanilla extract (1 teaspoon)

- Baking soda (1/4 teaspoon)

- Almond cup (half cup)

- A pinch of salt

- Trivia (9 packets)

How to Prepare your Chocolate Keto Brownies?

1. The very first thing that you need to do is preheat the microwave to 375 degrees Fahrenheit.

2. Take a bowl and mix the eggs, almond milk, cream cheese, vanilla extract, and coconut oil and stir it well until smooth.

3. Take another bowl and mix the almond flour, cocoa powder, baking soda, trivia, salt and coconut flour and add the wet ingredients into it and stir it well.

4. Finally, the pour the entire batter into a pan and bake for at least half an hour. Once it is out, let it cool for 5 minutes and then cut, as you desire.

How You Give It a Personal Touch

You can serve it with a whipped heavy cream or even add caramel and Walden farms butterscotch. In fact, you can also prepare a vanilla frosting and serve the brownies. Adding these ingredients to the brownies will simply accentuate the whole recipe and your guests will be in praise for your culinary skills.

Try making this easy and simple recipe at home and there won't be any need to order brownies from bakery shops. Whether it is a get-together or a you simply feel like eating brownies, this recipe is an apt consideration.

HOW TO PREPARE YOUR KETO PIE CRUST

Ingredients With Nutritional Information

- 2 cups of almond flour (192grams of almond flour) – 94g of fat, 1100 total calories

- 4 tablespoons of butter – 46grams of fat, 407 total calories

- 2 large eggs- 10grams of fat, 150 total calories

- 1 teaspoon salt- 0 grams of fat and 0 calories

- Take a medium size mixing bowl, place the almond flour and mix well with butter.

- Add the eggs and salt and continue to mix thoroughly until the dough comes together.

- Try to make it as a ball pulling it from the edge of the bowl.

- Add a little more of almond flour if the mixture is sticky and mix it up until you get a consistent mixture that can be rolled out.

- Place the dough ball between two parchment papers and roll it into a 10" x 16" rectangle with a thickness of about ¼ inch.

How to Prepare Little Tart Shells

1. Cut circles into the dough to make miniature tarts.

2. Prepare the miniature cupcake pans with miniature cupcake papers.

3. Take out the dough circles carefully and press them into the paper cup. Use a Mini Tart Shaper to avoid unnecessary breakings.

4. Bake at 350 degrees F for about 5-6 minutes or until edges turn gold.

Despite all the simple ingredients used to make this ketogenic dessert, it is rich with fat and proteins. It immediately triggers the fat burning process in your body which you will almost sense. Ketogenic desserts do not only offer a fat burning solution but also a number of other health benefits such as lowering the risk of high blood pressure and reducing blood sugar and insulin levels. Why are you still waiting? Go, grab the pans and start cooking right now!

THE KETOGENIC WAFFLES OF PUMPKIN

Waffles are the best snacks, but they are quite high in calorie, so the dieticians, always advice not to eat it while following a diet plan as extra fat can be added to the body. But with the advent of new age cooking methods there are good fat free recipes, and the ketogenic waffles of pumpkin are one of the tasty food of the ketogenic diet plan.

Pumpkin is a very good vegetable, which can also be used as a fruit. The recipes of pumpkin are always good to eat and also to digest. The ketogenic waffles of pumpkin have the proper adequate measure resulting in a good low carbs diet waffle changing the face and taste of the waffle to a next level. The body builders who have tried this recipe are satisfied with not only the taste but also. the nutritional value it gives. The ketogenic waffles of pumpkin is a now a rage among all the diet lovers around the globe.

Ingredients:

- 6 to 7 tablespoons of flaxseed meal
- 8 tablespoons of pure almond meal
- 2 to 3 eggs
- 6 tablespoons of unsweetened thick coconut

milk

- 1 ½ tablespoons butter or saturated white oil

- 3 tablespoons of pure pumpkin puree

Method of Making the Ketogenic Waffles

1. 1.To make tasty ketogenic waffles of pumpkin you have to first measure all the ingredients properly and keep them aside.

2. Then you take a big bowl and mix the entire ingredients one after the other, resulting into a thick proportionate mixture.

3. Do check that the mixture should not be too light or too heavy or else it will get stuck in the waffle iron while cooking. Then make one time each of a waffle in the waffle iron.

4. Finally serve them hot with honey, which is very healthy.

THE NUTRITIONAL VALUE

The ketogenic waffle of pumpkin is high in all the nutrition's, as it not only get the taste of the butter and flour but also the added puree of the pumpkin gives it a different nutritional value for vegetable and ironic food method. It is also important that the ketogenic waffles are always served hot so that the food value does not miss in the recipe. The nutritional values chart is as follows

Calories -243: Fat – 189: Total Fat – 21.0g: Saturated Fat – 9.0g: Trans Fat – 0.0g: Cholesterol – 93mg: Sodium – 69mg: Potassium – 283mg: Total Carbohydrates – 4.9g: Dietary Fiber – 6.3g: Sugars – 1.8g Protein – 9.0g: Vitamin A 41%: Vitamin C 2% :Calcium 8% : Iron 11%

So the following nutritional value of the ketogenic waffle of pumpkin is balanced on all the food values. So now when you are planning to make a ketogenic waffle of pumpkin, just follow the steps and you would get a very tasty and healthy ketogenic waffle.

Further research shows that the ketogenic waffle are now made all over the world in many restaurants who are preparing and serving health foods, but these are only made when customers give special orders. The taste and value of food in hundred percent and the health is fully maintained without any fail. So now just follow the steps and methods and eat and enjoy tasty waffles in your diet plan without any thought or tension of extra fat, with the recipe of the ketogenic waffle of pumpkin at your platter.

Eating a well-balanced diet is very important to live a happy and healthy life. However, when eating low-carb, you should also know the significance of eating a sufficient amount of healthy fats. Fortunately, eggs are both high-fat and low-carb, yet by including some extra flavors and avocado or tomato for a deliciously smooth texture and extra fats, you can prepare Keto Mexican Scrambled Eggs for a proper meal that hits high notes of a low-carb diet. Adding chili can also be a very good addition as well as gives the recipe a delicious kick, it also helps in digestion and is packed full of vitamin C and can help to relieve headaches and muscle pains. Make scrambled eggs more energizing with the Keto Mexican Scrambled Eggs. Such a delicious breakfast will definitely satisfy your hunger and makes you happy.

Why Include Eggs in Your Breakfast?

Eggs are one of the most beneficial and most versatile foods on earth. One egg contains less than 1 gram of carbs and less than 6 grams of protein, making eggs a perfect food for a ketogenic lifestyle. Also, eggs have been shown to trigger the hormones that enhance the feeling of fullness and keep glucose levels stable, prompting lower calorie intakes for as long as 24 hours.

It is vital to eat the whole egg, as a large portion of an egg's nutrients are found in the yolk. The antioxidants, zeaxanthin, and lutein help to protect the health of the eye. In spite of the fact that egg yolks are high in cholesterol, devouring them does not raise the level of blood cholesterol in most of the people. The fact is eggs seem to modify LDL shape in a way that lessens the danger of heart diseases.

HOW TO MAKE KETO MEXICAN SCRAMBLED EGGS?

Here is a delicious recipe for making Keto Mexican Scrambled Eggs.

Keto Mexican Scrambled Eggs:

Make scrambled eggs more energizing with the Keto Mexican Scrambled Eggs. Such a delicious breakfast will definitely satisfy your hunger and makes you happy.

Ingredients

- 6 Eggs
- 1 Scallion
- 2 Jalapenos finely chopped pickled
- 1 Tomato finely chopped
- 3 oz Shredded cheese
- 2 tbsp Butter for frying
- Black pepper
- Salt

Instructions

1. Chop the jalapenos, tomatoes, and scallions

very finely.

2. Fry these in butter for 2 to 3 minutes on medium flame.

3. Beat the eggs and pour into pan.

4. Scramble the eggs for 2 minutes and add cheese and seasonings. Enjoy it!

This delicious Mexican scrambled eggs mean there truly is no reason for not having a deliciously prepared breakfast even on the busy mornings. Keto Mexican Scrambled Eggs is ready to serve. Enjoy your delicious Keto Mexican Scrambled Eggs.

KETO LASAGNA RECIPE FROM ITALIAN KITCHEN

The Ingredients Required

As the first thing, let's take a look at the ingredients that you will need to have in order to get started with preparing this recipe.

Ingredients

- For the meat sauce, you will need to get
- 1 lb mild Italian sausage
- 1 lb ground beef
- 1 small chopped onion
- 30 oz crushed tomatoes
- 4 garlic cloves

In order to prepare noodles, you will need to get

- 3 cups Mozzarella Cheese
- 8 oz Cream cheese
- ½ cup Parmesan cheese
- 1 tsp Granulated onion and granulated garlic each
- 4 Eggs

To complete the cheese filling, you can get

- 5 cups Mozzarella cheese

- ½ cup full fat Ricotta cheese

- ½ cup Parmesan cheese

Instructions

1. As the first thing, you should know how you are going to prepare meat sauce. To do that, you should cook sausage and ground beef at a medium temperature. (You are doing this with the objective of removing excessive fat in the food.)

2. Then you can add garlic and tomato and mix the ingredients. After mixing for some time, you can add water along with water if required.

3. Now you need to bring the mixture to a slimmer and let it stay for a couple of hours after reducing the heat.

4. Once meat sauce is prepared, you will be able to go ahead with the preparation of noodles. You need to take a large bowl in order to do that. In the large bowl, you must combine cream cheese, eggs and Italian seasoning.

5. To the same mixture, you will need to add onion and garlic as well. You can take a hand

mixer and mix it for a couple of minutes. Once you feel that the mixture has become smooth, you can stop mixing.

6. Then you should fold Parmesan and Mozzarella cheese and add to the mixture. The mixture should then be laid on top of a cookie sheet and kept inside an oven that is heated for a temperature of 375 degrees Fahrenheit. You should keep it for a period of about 30 minutes.

Now you have come to the final, but most important step, which is about building the lasagna.

7. You need to pour meat sauce that you have prepared into a casserole dish. Then you need to add a noodles layer. You must repeat this process for one more time. But you need to put noodles first.

8. Once you complete adding the second layer of Mozzarella Cheese, you need to add another layer of sauce. The top should be filled with remaining sauce and noodles.

9. You should now place lasagna inside a preheated oven. The temperature should be 375 degrees Fahrenheit. You will need to bake your lasagna for a period of around 45 minutes. When you see that it has become bubbly, you can take out of the oven.

10. add the remaining amounts of Parmesan cheese and Mozzarella cheese you have to the top. After doing that, you should bake it for another 20 minutes.

11. Then you can let cheese melt and turn into golden brown color. Once it is done, you can keep lasagna for 15 minutes and enjoy it.

SLOW COKER FRITTA

Ingredients:

- 8 large eggs
- 1 lb. 80/20 Ground Beef, browned
- 5 oz. Mozzarella Cheese
- 2 oz. Parmesan
- 1 medium Bell Pepper
- 1 tsp. Onion Powder
- 1/2 tsp. Garlic Powder
- 2 tsp. Chili Powder
- 5 oz. Spinach
- 1/2 tsp. Cumin
- 1/4 tsp. Cayenne Pepper
- 1/4 cup Salsa
- 1/4 cup Sour Cream
- Salt and Pepper to Taste

Instructions:

1. In a pan over medium heat, brown the ground beef. After one side browns, add chopped bell pepper and spinach.

2. Meanwhile mix together eggs, spices, and 2/3 of the cheese.

3. Add egg mixture to a grease slow cooker, and then add the beef to that

4. Slowly stir to combine all of the ingredients, then top with remaining 1/3 cheese.

5. Cook on low for 2-3 hours or until eggs are firm

BISCUITS & SAUSAGE GRAVY

Ingredients:

Biscuit:

- 1 cup Almond Flour
- 1/4 cup Coconut Flour
- 1/4 cup Butter
- 2 tbsp. Sour Cream
- 1 tsp. Baking Powder
- 1/4 tsp. Salt
- Sausage Gravy:
- 1 1/2 cup Heavy Cream
- 1/2 tsp. Guar Gum
- 1/2 lb. Breakfast Sausage
- Salt and Pepper to Taste

This makes 4 servings. Each serving:

- 590.3 Calories
- 54.3 Fats (g)
- Net Carbs (g)
- 16.0 Protein (g)

Instructions:

1. Combine all ingredients for the biscuits, then set aside.

2. Brown sausage in a pan over medium-high heat. Once finished, add to the slow cooker.

3. Add heavy cream and salt and pepper to the sausage. Then, add guar gum and whisk together.

4. Roll out biscuits and place on top of the sausage gravy.

5. Cook on high for 2 hours.

BREAKFAST PIE

Ingredients:

- 1/2 cup Almond Flour
- 1/2 cup Parmesan Cheese
- 12 oz. Daikon Radish, grated
- 1 lb. Breakfast Sausage
- 1/2 Red Bell Pepper
- 8 Large Eggs
- 2 tsp. Dried Parsley
- 2 tsp. Dried Basil
- 1 tsp. Onion Powder
- 1 tsp. Garlic Powder
- Salt and Pepper to Taste

Instructions:

1. Grate daikon radish into a bowl. Dice red bell pepper and set aside.

2. Add all ingredients to daikon radish and mix together well.

3. Grease slow cooker with butter or cooking spray, then pour all ingredients in.

4. Set on low for 6-8 hours, and then use a spatula to remove the breakfast pie from the slow cooker.

5. Slice into 6 servings.

ZUCCHINI BAKED GREEN APPLES

Ingredients:

- 12 oz. Zucchini
- 3/4 cup Water
- 1 packet Sugar-Free Lime (or Lemon) Jello
- 1 tbsp. Cinnamon
- 1 tsp. Nutmeg
- 2 tbsp. Xylitol
- 1/2 cup Heavy Cream

This makes 4 servings. Each serving:

- 148.0 Calories
- 12.5 Fats (g)
- Net Carbs (g)
- 2.0 Protein (g)

Instructions:

1. Peel zucchini and slice into 1/6" pieces. Using a mandolin will help with speed.

2. Add all ingredients (except heavy cream) to a slow cooker, and then stir together.

3. Cook on low for 2 1/2 hours.

4. Add 1/2 cup heavy cream and gently mix into the sauce.

ARMADILLO EGGS

Ingredients:

- 1 lb. Ground Pork
- 1/4 cup Almond Flour
- 2 tbsp. Parmesan Cheese
- 2 tsp. Chili Powder
- 1 tsp. Garlic Powder
- 1/2 tsp. Onion Powder
- 1/4 tsp. Red Pepper Flakes
- 7 small Jalapenos
- 3 oz. Cream Cheese
- Salt and Pepper to Taste

This makes 3 servings. Each serving:

- 590.3 Calories
- 49.0 Fats (g)
- 3.8 Net Carbs (g)
- 32.0 Protein (g)

Instructions:

1. Mix ground pork with all spices, set aside.

2. Chop jalapeno peppers in half, and then de-seed them by scraping innards out with a spoon.

3. Fill half jalapeno pepper with cream cheese, and then replace the other half on top. Repeat.

4. Wrap each jalapeno with the pork mixture.

5. Set all armadillo eggs in the slow cooker and cook for 5 hours on low.

Optional: Top with additional bacon bits and cheese.

CHEESEBURGER MEATBALLS

Ingredients:

- 1 lb. Ground Beef (80/20)
- 12-18 Cheese Cubes (depending on size of meatballs)
- 1/4 cup Almond Flour
- 1 large Egg
- 3/4 tsp. Garlic
- 1/2 tsp. Onion Powder
- 1/4 tsp. Cumin
- 1 tsp. Worcestershire Sauce
- Salt and Pepper to Taste

This makes 5 servings. Each serving:

- 500.0 Calories
- 40.0 Fats (g)
- 1.2 Net Carbs (g)
- 32.0 Protein (g)

Instructions:

1. Combine all ingredients (except for cheese) into a bowl. Mix together well.

2. Form meatballs with cheese cubes in the center, making sure there are no holes left in the meatball mixture.

3. Place all meatballs into the slow cooker and cook for 5 hours on low, or 3 hours on high.

Note: Putting them on high for 30 minutes, then turning to low helps seal the meatballs and helps keep the cheese inside.

CHEESEBURGER PIE

Ingredients:

- 1 lb. Ground Beef, browned with fat drained
- 1/4 cup Mayonnaise
- 4 oz. Cream Cheese
- 8 oz. Cheddar Cheese
- 2 large Eggs
- 1 tsp. Dried Minced Onion
- 1 cube Beef Bouillon Cube, crumbled
- 1/4 tsp. Onion Powder
- 1/4 tsp. Garlic Powder
- Salt and Pepper to Taste

This makes 6 servings. Each serving:

- 401.5 Calories
- 32.5 Fats (g)
- 1.7 Net Carbs (g)
- 24.3 Protein (g)

Instructions:

1. Grate cheddar cheese, separating half of it for

later.

2. Mix all ingredients together in a bowl (except for half of the cheese).

3. Press all ingredients into a greased slow cooker.

4. Top with cheese and turn on low for 4-5 hours or high for 3 hours.

5. Garnish with ketchup, mayonnaise, and pickles.

CHEESY SAUSAGE & MUSHROOM SOUP

Ingredients:

Starting:

- 12 oz. Andouille Sausage, sliced thin
- 9 oz. Baby Bella Mushrooms, sliced thin
- 1 tbsp. Olive Oil
- 1/4 cup Butter
- 1/2 medium Onion, diced
- 1 tsp. Garlic, minced
- 3 cups Chicken Stock
- 1 tsp. Guar Gum
- 1/8 tsp. Nutmeg

Finishing:

- 1 cup Heavy Cream
- 8 oz. Cheddar Cheese, shredded
- Salt and Pepper to Taste

This makes 6 servings. Each serving:

- 558.2 Calories

- 50.2 Fats (g)

- Net Carbs (g)

- 23.5 Protein (g)

Instructions:

1. In a pan over medium high heat, brown sausage until cooked. Set aside.

2. In the same pan, cook onion and mushroom in the pan until soft.

3. Add stock, nutmeg, garlic and guar gum into the slow cooker and whisk together until guar gum is incorporated.

4. Add the sausage, onion, mushrooms, and butter into the slow cooker and mix together.

5. Cook on low for 4 hours or high for 3 hours. Once finished, add the finishing ingredients and stir together.

6. Cook for an additional 30 minutes on high without the lid in the slow cooker.

CHICKEN BACON RANCH CASSEROLE

Ingredients:

Starting:

- 5 Chicken Thighs, deboned (~1 3/4 lbs.)
- 8 slices Bacon
- 8 oz. Broccoli Florets
- 8 oz. Cheddar Cheese, grated
- 1/2 cup Ranch Dressing
- 1 tsp. Onion Powder
- 1 tsp. Garlic Powder
- Salt and Pepper to Taste

Finishing:

- 1 tbsp. Dried Parsley
- 1/2 tsp. Dried Dill Weed
- 1/2 tsp. Dried Basil

This makes 8 servings. Each serving:

- 507.5 Calories
- 42.1 Fats (g)

- 2.5 Net Carbs (g)
- 27.8 Protein (g)

Instructions:

1. Debone chicken thighs using kitchen shears.
2. Place all ingredients in the slow cooker and mix together.
3. Cook on low for 5 hours, or high for 3 hours.
4. Mix everything together, shredding the chicken as you stir. Add finishing herbs and mix again.
5. Optionally remove the lid and cook for another 30 minutes to reduce.

CHICKEN CHILI

Ingredients:

- 5 Chicken Thighs, deboned
- 3 cups Chicken Broth
- 1 tbsp. Butter
- 1 medium Jalapeno Pepper, minced1 medium Jalapeno Pepper, minced
- 1 medium Green Pepper, chopped
- 2 Green Onions, chopped1 tbsp. Ground Cumin
- 1 1/2 tsp. Ground Coriander
- 1 tsp. Ancho Chili Powder
- 1 tsp. Garlic Powder
- 1/2 tsp. Onion Powder
- Juice 1 Lime
- 1/4 cup Cilantro Leaves, chopped
- Salt and Pepper to Taste

This makes 4 servings. Each serving:

- 476.3 Calories
- 33.3 Fats (g)

- 3.6 Net Carbs (g)
- 34.8 Protein (g)

Instructions:

1. Debone chicken thighs using kitchen shears.

2. Add all ingredients to the slow cooker and mix together until seasoning is well distributed.

3. Cook on low for 5 hours, or high for 3 hours.

4. As an option, you can turn this into a rich white chicken chili by adding 1/2 cup heavy cream at the end.

CHICKEN SWEDISH

Meatballs

Ingredients:

Meatball:

- 1 lb Ground Chicken Thigh
- 1/4 cup Almond Flour
- 1/4 cup Flaxseed Meal
- 1 large Egg
- 1/4 tsp. Allspice
- 1/4 tsp. Nutmeg
- Salt and Pepper to Taste

Starting:

- 1 1/2 cups Chicken Stock
- 1/2 cup Sour Cream
- 2 tbsp. Butter
- 1 tbsp. Soy Sauce
- 1/2 tsp. Guar Gum

Finishing:

- 1/2 cup Heavy Cream

- 1/2 tsp. Guar Gum

This makes 4 servings. Each serving:

- 471.5 Calories
- 36.8 Fats (g)
- 2.9 Net Carbs (g)
- 28.3 Protein (g)

GENERAL TSO'S MEATBALLS

Ingredients:

<u>Sauce:</u>

- 1 cup Beef Broth
- 2 tbsp. Soy Sauce
- 2 tbsp. Rice Vinegar
- 4 tbsp. Sugar Free Maple Syrup (Such as Walden Farm's)
- 2 tbsp. Chili Garlic Paste
- 1 tsp. Garlic Powder
- 1 tsp. Onion powder
- 1 tsp. Ancho Chili Powder
- 1 tsp. Ginger Powder
- 1/4 tsp. Cayenne Pepper
- 1/2 tsp. Guar Gum

<u>Meatballs:</u>

- 1 lb. Ground Beef
- 1/4 cup Flaxseed Meal
- 1 large Egg

- 1 tsp. Garlic Powder

- 1 tsp. Ginger Powder

- 1 tsp. Onion Powder

- 1 tsp. Sesame Oil

- 2 tsp. Sesame Seeds

- Salt and Pepper to Taste

This makes 4 servings. Each serving:

- 374.0 Calories

- 27.8 Fats (g)

- 2.4 Net Carbs (g)

- 24.8 Protein (g)

Instructions:

1. Mix together all of the sauce ingredients in slow cooker. Use a whisk to incorporate the guar gum.

2. Mix together all meatball ingredients, and then form into meatballs. About 18 in total.

3. Place meatballs in the slow cooker and cook on low for 5 hours or high for 3 hours.

4. Remove the lid and cook on high for 1 hour. Remove meatballs from sauce and use an immersion blender to emulsify sauce.

163

5. Serve meatballs with sauce spooned over the top.

SPANISH MEATBALLS

Ingredients:

Meatballs:

- 1 lb. Ground Pork
- 1/4 cup Shelled Hemp Hearts
- 1 large Egg
- 1 tsp. Minced Garlic
- 1/2 tsp. Onion Powder
- 2 tsp. Paprika
- 1/2 tsp. Dried Thyme
- Salt and Pepper to Taste

Sauce:

- 1/2 cup Canned Tomatoes with Jalapenos
- 1/4 cup Heavy Cream
- 1/2 tsp. Guar Gum

This makes 4 servings. Each serving:

- 444.3 Calories
- 35.8 Fats (g)

- 2.3 Net Carbs (g)
- 24.3 Protein (g)

Instructions

1. Mix together all meatball ingredients in a bowl. Set aside.

2. Add all sauce ingredients to the slow cooker, then whisk together thoroughly to incorporate guar gum.

3. Roll out meatballs and place in the bottom of the slow cooker, about 18 in total.

4. Cook on low for 5-6 hours or high for 4 hours.

5. Remove meatballs from the slow cooker and set aside. Use an immersion blender o emulsify the sauce.

6. Serve sauce spooned over meatballs.

HONEY SESAME CHICKEN

Ingredients:

<u>Sauce:</u>

- 1/4 cup Erythritol
- 1/4 cup Rice Vinegar
- 2 tbsp. Reduced Sugar Ketchup
- 1 tbsp. Soy Sauce
- 1/2 tsp. Mango Extract
- 1/2 tsp. Guar Gum
- 7 drops Liquid Stevia

<u>Starting:</u>

- 4 Chicken Thighs
- 1 tsp. Garlic Powder
- 1 tsp. Toasted Sesame Seeds
- Salt and Pepper to Taste

<u>Finishing:</u>

- 1/4 tsp. Guar Gum
- 1 tbsp. Reduced Sugar Ketchup
- 1 tbsp. Soy Sauce

- 1 tbsp. Erythritol

- 2 tbsp. Rice Wine Vinegar

- Juice 1/2 Lemon

This makes 5 servings. Each serving:

- 399.8 Calories

- 27.8 Fats (g)

- 1.3 Net Carbs (g)

- 32.8 Protein (g)

Instructions:

1. Whisk all sauce ingredients together in the bottom of the slow cooker until guar gum is incorporated.

2. Add all starting ingredients to the slow cooker.

3. Cook on low for 6-7 hours, or high for 5 hours.

4. Once finished, add all finishing ingredients and shred chicken using a fork. Mix everything together.

5. Serve on lettuce as lettuce wraps, or as a meal over vegetables.

LAMB KOFTA

Ingredients:

<u>Kofta:</u>

- 1 lb. Ground Lamb
- 1/4 Red Onion
- 1/4 cup Mint Leaves, chopped
- 2 tsp. Garlic, minced
- 2 tsp. Paprika
- 1 tsp. Dried Parsley
- 1 tsp. Cumin
- 1/2 tsp. Coriander
- 1/2 tsp. Allspice

<u>Sauce:</u>

- Fat from Slow Cooker
- 1/2 cup Full Fat Yogurt
- 2 tbsp. TahiniJuice
- 1/2 LemonSalt to Taste
- 1/4 tsp. Cumin

This makes 4 servings. Each serving:

- 412.5 Calories
- 32.4 Fats (g)
- Net Carbs (g)
- 23.3 Protein (g)

Instructions:

1. Mix together all of the kofta ingredients and form into oval shaped meatballs.

2. Place in the bottom of the slow cooker and cook on low for 5-6 hours or high for 4 hours.

3. Once done, take meatballs out of the slow cooker and set aside.

4. Mix together all sauce ingredients and serve with kofta.

LEG OF LAMB

Ingredients:

- 3 1/2 lbs. Leg of Lamb, bone out
- 1/2 cup Olive Oil
- 1/2 cup Chicken Stock
- 1/4 cup Dry White Wine
- 1/4 cup White Wine Vinegar1 medium Lemon, Juice and Zest
- 4 tsp. Garlic, minced1 tsp. Dried Oregano
- 1 tsp. Nutmeg
- 2 tbsp. Fresh Mint, chopped Salt and Pepper to Taste

This makes 10 servings. Each serving:

- 445.0 Calories
- 38.2 Fats (g)
- 1.4 Net Carbs (g)
- 28.1 Protein (g)

Instructions:

1. Add leg of lamb to the bottom of the slow cooker.

2. Add the rest of the ingredients, pouring over the leg of lamb as you add them.

3. Cook on low for 6 hours.

4. Remove lamb from slow cooker and slice.

5. Serve with spooning of juice from the slow cooker.

MEXICAN PORK SHOULDER

Ingredients:

- 5-6 lb. Pork Butt (Boston Butt)
- 1 tbsp. Kosher Salt
- 1 tsp. Black Pepper
- 1 tbsp. Cumin
- 2 tsp. Coriander
- 1 tsp. Garlic Powder
- 1 tsp. Onion Powder
- 1/8 tsp. Cinnamon
- 1/2 cup Chicken StockJuice
- 1/2 lime

This makes 12 servings. Each serving:

- 423.3 Calories
- 29.5 Fats (g)
- 0.5 Net Carbs (g)
- 36.9 Protein (g)

Instructions:

1. Mix all spices together in a small bowl.

2. Sprinkle seasoning over pork butt until all sides are covered.

3. Pour chicken stock into the bottom of a slow cooker, then place pork butt inside.

4. Cook on low for 6 hours or high for 4 hours. Shred the pork into the juices and cook for another 1 hour on low.

5. Before serving, squeeze lime juice over pork

MOLE CHILI

Ingredients:

- 1 1/2 lbs. Ground Beef
- 2 tbsp. Olive Oil
- 2 tsp. Garlic Powder
- 1 tsp. Onion Powder
- 1/2 Red Bell pepper, chopped (1 medium)
- 1/2 Green Bell pepper, chopped (1 medium)
- 1 tbsp. Chili Powder1 tsp. Paprika
- 1 tsp. Dried Oregano
- 2 tsp. Ground Cumin
- 1/2 tsp. Cinnamon
- 1/4 cup White Wine
- 1/2 cup Tomatoes and Green Chile (from a can)
- 1/2 cup Green Olives, sliced
- 2 tbsp. Cocoa Powder
- 1/4 cup Reduced Sugar Ketchup
- 1/2 cup fresh Cilantro, chopped
- 2 Chilis in Adobo Sauce

- 2 medium Jalapenos, sliced

This makes 5 servings. Each serving:

- 463.8 Calories
- 35.4 Fats (g)
- Net Carbs (g)
- 24.6 Protein (g)

Instructions:

1. Over medium-high heat, brown ground beef in olive oil over the stove.

2. Once browned, transfer beef to the slow cooker. Then add all of the other ingredients.

3. Mix together well, and then cook on low for 6 hours or high for 4 hours.

PIZZA DIP

Ingredients:

White Sauce Pizza Dip

- 2 cups Mozzarella Cheese, Shredded (8 oz.)
- 1 1/4 cup Sour Cream (12 oz.)
- 1 cup Ricotta Cheese
- 1/4 cup Parmesan Cheese
- 1/4 medium Onion, diced
- 1 tbsp. Garlic, minced
- 1/4 cup Salsa
- 1/4 cup Mayonnaise
- 4 tsp. Italian Seasoning
- 1 6 oz. Package Pepperoni, sliced Salt and Pepper to taste

This makes 6 servings. Each serving:

- 511.5 Calories
- 43.3 Fats (g)
- Net Carbs (g)
- 21.7 Protein (g)

Instructions:

1. Prep all ingredients and meat by dicing and mincing.

2. Mix together all ingredients into a crock pot.

3. Cook on low for 3 hours.

POACHED SALMON

Ingredients:

- 1 cup Chicken Stock
- 1/2 cup Dry White Wine
- 1/4 tsp. Onion Powder
- 1/4 medium Lemon
- 1/2 tsp. Dried Dill Weed
- 1/2 tsp. Dried Tarragon Salt and Pepper to Taste
- 3 6 oz. Salmon Fillets

This makes 3 servings. Each serving:

- 324.7 Calories
- 13.7 Fats (g)
- 1.3 Net Carbs (g)
- 36.7 Protein (g)

Instructions:

1. Combine all ingredients (except for salmon) in a slow cooker. Squeeze the lemon juice into the slow cooker and leave the whole 1/4 remaining lemon in the broth.

2. Add salmon to the juices in the crock pot.

3. Cook on high for 20 minutes or until salmon is cooked through according to taste.

4. Optionally add 1/4 cup heavy cream and 2 tbsp. butter to the slow cooker. Use an immersion blender to create a sauce

THAI PEANUT CHICKEN

Ingredients:

- 5 small Chicken Thighs, deboned (~1 3/4 lbs.)
- 6 tbsp. Salsa
- 1/4 cup Soy Sauce
- 1 tbsp. Fish Sauce
- 2 tbsp. Rice Vinegar
- 1 tsp. Onion Powder
- 1 tsp. Garlic Powder
- 2 tsp. Ginger Powder
- 2 tbsp. Chili Garlic Paste
- 1/4 cup PB2 (Powdered Peanuts)Juice 1 Lime
- 1/2 cup Cilantro, chopped
- 1/4 cup Coconut Oil

This makes 5 servings. Each serving:

- 475.0 Calories
- 36.0 Fats (g)
- 2.8 Net Carbs (g)
- 31.8 Protein (g)

Instructions:

1. Debone chicken thighs using kitchen shears.

2. Place chicken thighs in the bottom of the slow cooker.

3. In a bowl, mix together all of the ingredients, then pour over the chicken. Use your hands to cover the chicken with the sauce.4. Cook on low for 5-6 hours, or high for 4 hours.

4. Remove lid and shred the chicken. Cook for another 60 minutes on low, or 30 minutes on high.

MAPLE PUDDING POKE CAKE

Ingredients:

Cake:

- 1 1/2 cup Almond Flour
- 2 tsp. Baking Powder
- 3/4 cup Erythritol
- 5 large Eggs
- 6 tbsp. Butter
- 1/4 tsp. Liquid Stevia
- 6 oz. Cream Cheese
- 1 tsp. Vanilla
- 2 tsp. Maple

Extract Topping:

- 1/2 cup Heavy Cream
- 1/3 cup Sugar Free Maple Syrup (Walden Farm's)
- 1/2 tsp. Guar Gum

This makes 8 servings. Each serving:

- 366.9 Calories

- 35.4 Fats (g)

- Net Carbs (g)

- Protein (g)

Instructions:

1. Mix together all of the dry cake ingredients. Using a hand mixer, mix together all of the wet cake ingredients.

2. Using a hand mixer, mix the dry ingredients into the wet.

3. Line a slow cooker with parchment paper, and then pour cake batter into the well.

4. Cook on low for 2 hours. Turn the slow cooker off and let cool for 30 minutes.

5. Remove cake from the slow cooker and carefully poke holes into the top using a fork.

6. Using a hand mixer, combine all topping ingredients until thickened. Pour over the top of the cake and let sit at least 10 minutes

PUMPKIN PIE CUSTARD

Ingredients:

- 15 oz. Canned Pumpkin
- 1 1/2 cups Heavy Cream
- 1/2 cup Xylitol
- 4 large Eggs
- 4 tbsp. Butter
- 1 tbsp. Vanilla
- 2 tsp. Cinnamon
- 1/2 tsp. Nutmeg
- 1/2 tsp. Ginger
- 1/4 tsp. Allspice
- 1/8 tsp. Clove

This makes 8 servings. Each serving:

- 366.9 Calories
- 35.4 Fats (g)
- Net Carbs (g)
- Protein (g)

Instructions:

1. Mix together all ingredients into a slow cooker.

2. Cook on low for 5-6 hours, or high for 4 hours.

3. Let cool for 30 minutes, and then use a serving spoon to dish out custard.

RASPBERRY SWIRL COFFEE CAKE

Ingredients:

<u>Cake:</u>

- 1 1/2 cup Almond Flour
- 2 tsp. Baking Powder
- 1/2 cup Erythritol
- 4 large Eggs6 tbsp. Butter
- 1/4 tsp. Liquid Stevia
- 1 tsp. VanillaRaspberry Swir
- l:2 oz. Raspberries4 oz. Cream Cheese
- 2 tbsp. Butter
- 2 tbsp. Erythritol
- 1/2 tsp. Vanilla

This makes 8 servings. Each serving:

- 310.4 Calories
- 29.0 Fats (g)
- Net Carbs (g)
- Protein (g)

Instructions:

1. Mix together the dry cake ingredients into a bowl. In a separate bowl, mix together the wet cake ingredients using a hand mixer.

2. Using a hand mixer, mix the dry cake ingredients into the wet. Set aside.

3. Using a hand mixer, mix together all of the raspberry swirl ingredients and set aside.

4. Line a slow cooker with parchment paper, then pour in the cake batter. Use a spatula to flatten the mixture out.

5. Spoon dollops of the raspberry swirl mixture on top of the batter, giving space in between each dollop.

6. Use a knife to swirl the raspberry mixture into the cake batter.

7. Cook on low for 2 1/2 hours.8. Turn slow cooker off and let cool for 30 minutes. Remove cake from slow cooker and slice.

SPICE CAKE

Ingredients:

<u>Cake:</u>

- 1 3/4 cups Almond Flour
- 1/2 cup Xylitol
- 1/4 tsp. Stevia
- 2 tsp Baking Powder
- 1/2 cup Salted Butter, melted
- 5 large Eggs
- 1/2 cup Coconut Milk, unsweetened
- 1/4 cup Sour Cream
- 1 tsp Vanilla Extract
- 3 tbsp. Psyllium Husk Powder
- 1 tsp. Cinnamon
- 1 tsp. Ground Ginger
- 1/2 tsp. Nutmeg
- 1/2 tsp.

<u>All spice Frosting:</u>

- 10 oz. Cream Cheese

- 10 tbsp. Butter

- 3 tbsp. Heavy Cream

- 1/4 cup Xylitol

- 1/4 tsp. Stevia Juice

- 1/2 lemon

This makes 12 servings. Each serving:

- 420.9 Calories

- 37.6 Fats (g)

- Net Carbs (g)

- Protein (g)

Instructions:

1. Mix together all dry cake ingredients into a bowl. In a separate bowl, mix together all of the wet cake ingredients.

2. Using a hand mixer, mix all dry cake ingredients into the wet until well incorporated.

3. Line bottom of slow cooker with parchment paper, then pour in cake batter. Spread smooth with a spatula.

4. Cook on low for 2 1/2 hours, then turn off and remove lid. Let cool for 30 minutes.

5. While cake is cooling, use a hand mixer to mix together all of the frosting ingredients.

6. Once cake is cool, remove from the slow cooker and frost

BROWNIES

Ingredients:

- 1 1/4 cups Almond Flour
- 2 tbsp. Dutch Process Cocoa Powder, unsweetened
- 8 tbsp. Butter, melted
- 2 tsp. Vanilla Extract
- 1/2 tsp. Coffee Extract (optional)
- 3/4 cup Xylitol
- 2 large Eggs
- 2 large Egg Yolks
- 3/4 cup Sugar Free Chocolate Chips (112g)
- 1/4 tsp. Salt

This makes 12 servings. Each serving:

- 224.9 Calories
- 17.5 Fats (g)
- Net Carbs (g)
- Protein (g)

Instructions:

1. Add all ingredients (except for chocolate chips) into a bowl and mix together using a hand mixer.

2. Once a thick batter is formed, fold in chocolate chips. Set aside.

3. Line the bottom of a slow cooker with parchment paper, then spread the batter out evenly.

4. Cook on low for 2 hours.5. Let cool for 15 minutes, and then remove from the slow cooker. Slice into 14 and serve.

CONCLUSION

It is important that you conduct a complete research to assure that the keto diet you are following is reliable and will help you maintain the nutrient level of your body. You have to assure that you maintain your diet plan and stay committed to what you are having. That is the only way you can stay in ketosis and assure that you enjoy all the healthy benefits that come with the diet plan.

Many individuals start the diet plan without knowing about the dangers of the keto diet. This is the reason when they are unable to maintain the diet plan properly they have to deal with various side effects that come with the process. This is the reason instead of losing weight they have to deal with other health problems that make them gain weight once again. That is why it is advised that before you can get started with the keto diet, it is important that you study the diet plan, process and dangers of the keto diet properly. That is the only way you will know whether you should start the diet plan or not. Another important thing that you have to consider doing is consulting your doctor.

In case you are dealing with some health issues, going on a keto diet can be dangerous for your body. Ask your doctor whether you can go on a keto diet or not. He will explain all the dangers of the keto diet associated with your health condition and help you decide whether it is the right option for you or not. If you are on a keto diet and notice some reactions, it is better that you stop the diet plan and consult an expert.

DISCLAIMER

The information contained within this eBook is strictly for educational purposes. If you wish to apply ideas contained in this eBook, you are taking full responsibility for your actions.

The author has made every effort to ensure the accuracy of the information within this book was correct at time of publication. The author does not assume and hereby disclaims any liability to any party for any loss, damage, or disruption caused by errors or omissions, whether such errors or omissions result from accident, negligence, or any other cause. (DIET, Intermittent fasting)

Do not go yet;
One last thing to do

If you enjoyed this book or found it useful, I'd be very grateful if you'd post a short review on it. Your support really does make a difference and I read all the reviews personally so I can get your feedback and make this book even better.

Thanks again for your support!